support type 1 diabetes for adults

MENU

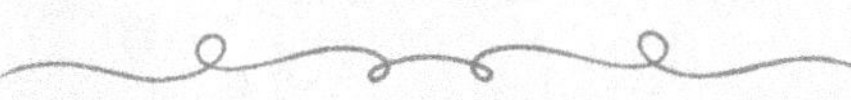

BREAKFAST

MENU

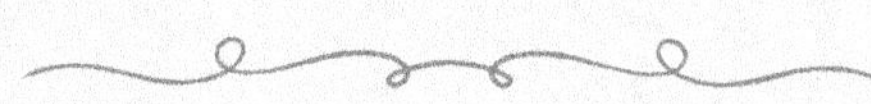

LUNCH

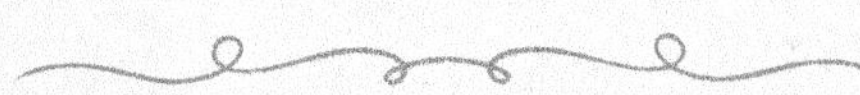

MENU

DINNER

MENU

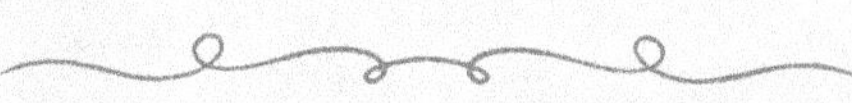

SNACKS

MENU

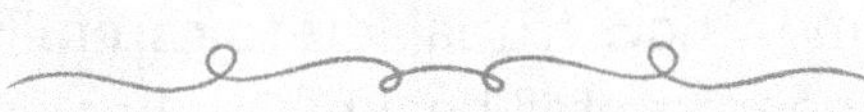

DESSERTS

Introduction

Welcome to the "Type 1 Diabetes Cookbook for Adults." This book is designed with you in mind, aiming to make managing type 1 diabetes both straightforward and enjoyable. As someone living with type 1 diabetes, you know how crucial it is to carefully manage your diet to keep your blood sugar levels stable and support overall health. Our goal is to provide you with a collection of delicious, easy-to-prepare recipes that fit seamlessly into your lifestyle while supporting your diabetes management goals.

Understanding Type 1 Diabetes
Type 1 diabetes is an autoimmune condition where the body's immune system mistakenly attacks insulin-producing beta cells in the pancreas. This results in little to no insulin production, requiring individuals to administer insulin externally to regulate blood sugar levels. Unlike type 2 diabetes, which is often associated with lifestyle factors, type 1 diabetes is usually diagnosed in children or young adults and is a lifelong condition.

Managing Blood Sugar Levels
Effective management of type 1 diabetes involves a combination of insulin therapy, regular blood glucose monitoring, and a balanced diet. Carbohydrates play a significant role in blood sugar levels, so understanding how they impact your body is essential. This cookbook provides a variety of recipes with controlled carbohydrate content to help you maintain stable blood glucose levels throughout the day.

The Role of Diet in Diabetes Management
Diet is a cornerstone of diabetes management. By focusing on nutrient-dense foods, you can support your overall health while keeping your blood sugar levels in check. This cookbook emphasizes balanced meals that include a mix of lean proteins, healthy fats, and complex carbohydrates. Each recipe is crafted to provide a satisfying meal without causing spikes in blood glucose levels.

We've included practical tips and nutritional information to help you make informed choices. Whether you're preparing a quick breakfast, a hearty lunch, or a satisfying dinner, you'll find recipes that are both flavorful and diabetes-friendly. Additionally, we've included sections on snacks and desserts that are designed to satisfy your cravings without compromising your health goals.

As you explore these recipes, remember that managing type 1 diabetes is a personal journey. What works for one person may not work for another, so we encourage you to use this cookbook as a guide and adapt recipes to fit your individual needs and preferences.

Thank you for choosing this cookbook as a resource in your diabetes management journey. We hope that the recipes and tips inside will help you enjoy a vibrant, balanced lifestyle while effectively managing your condition.
Here's to your health and well-being!

1. Spinach and Feta Omelet

Ingredients:

- 3 eggs
- 1 tbsp butter or olive oil
- 1 cup fresh spinach, chopped
- 2 tbsp crumbled feta cheese
- Salt and pepper to taste

Breakfast

PreparationTime: 5 minutes
Cook Time: 5-7 minutes
Total Time: 10-12 minutes
Serves: 1

↓↓↓

1. Crack the eggs into a small bowl and beat them lightly with a fork until blended.

2. Heat a small non-stick skillet over medium heat and melt the butter or heat the olive oil.

3. Pour the eggs into the skillet and let them sit for 20-30 seconds to set the bottom.

4. Use a spatula to gently push the cooked egg towards the center, tilting the pan to allow the uncooked egg to flow to the edges.

5. When the eggs are mostly set but still a bit runny on top, sprinkle the chopped spinach and crumbled feta over half of the omelet.

6. Use the spatula to fold the unfilled half of the omelet over the filled half.

7. Slide the folded omelet onto a plate and season with salt and pepper to taste.

8. Serve hot and enjoy!

2. Greek Yogurt with Berries and Chia Seeds

Ingredients:

- 1 cup plain Greek yogurt
- 1/2 cup mixed berries
 (such as blueberries, raspberries, blackberries)
- 1 tbsp chia seeds
- 1 tsp honey (optional)

Breakfast

PreparationTime: 5 minutes
Total Time: 5 minutes
Serves: 1

↓↓

1. Scoop the Greek yogurt into a bowl or serving dish.

2. Top the yogurt with the mixed berries.

3. Sprinkle the chia seeds over the top.

4. If desired, drizzle the honey over the top.

5. Serve immediately and enjoy!

The Greek yogurt provides protein, the berries add antioxidants and natural sweetness, and the chia seeds offer fiber, protein and healthy omega-3 fatty acids. This makes for a nutritious and delicious breakfast or snack.

3. Avocado and Egg Breakfast Bowl

Ingredients:

- 1 medium avocado, halved and pitted
- 2 large eggs
- 1 tbsp olive oil
- 1 tbsp chopped fresh cilantro (optional)
- Salt and pepper to taste

Breakfast

PreparationTime: 10 minutes
Cook Time: 5 minutes
Total Time: 15 minutes
Serves: 1

↓↓↓

1. In a small non-stick skillet, heat the olive oil over medium heat.

2. Crack the eggs into the skillet and cook for 2-3 minutes, or until the whites are set but the yolks are still runny.

3. Carefully transfer the cooked eggs to one of the avocado halves.

4. Sprinkle the eggs with a pinch of salt and pepper.

5. If desired, top with the chopped cilantro.

6. Serve the avocado and egg bowl immediately.

Nutrition Information (per serving):
- Calories: 320
- Total Carbs: 12g
- Fiber: 7g
- Net Carbs: 5g
- Protein: 12g
- Fat: 27g

This breakfast bowl is a great option for adults with type 1 diabetes as it is high in healthy fats from the avocado, moderate in carbs, and provides a good source of protein from the eggs. The healthy fats and protein can help stabilize blood sugar levels. Be sure to adjust insulin dosage accordingly.

4. Low-Carb Pancakes with Fresh Fruit

Ingredients:

Breakfast

- 3 large eggs
- 1/4 cup unsweetened almond milk
- 1 tbsp coconut flour
- 1 tbsp ground flaxseed
- 1 tsp baking powder
- 1/4 tsp ground cinnamon
- 1/4 tsp vanilla extract
- 1 cup mixed fresh berries (such as raspberries, blueberries, strawberries)
- Sugar-free maple syrup (optional)

PreparationTime: 10 minutes
Cook Time: 10-12 minutes
Total Time: 20-22 minutes
Serves: 2 (3 pancakes per serving)

↓↓

1. In a medium bowl, whisk together the eggs and almond milk until well combined.

2. Add the coconut flour, ground flaxseed, baking powder, cinnamon, and vanilla extract. Whisk until a smooth batter forms.

3. Heat a non-stick skillet or griddle over medium heat. Lightly grease with butter or non-stick cooking spray.

4. Scoop about 1/4 cup of the batter onto the hot surface, forming 3-inch pancakes. Cook for 2-3 minutes per side, or until golden brown.

5. Serve the low-carb pancakes warm, topped with the fresh mixed berries. Drizzle with a small amount of sugar-free maple syrup if desired.

Nutrition Information (per serving):
- Calories: 220
- Total Carbs: 12g
- Fiber: 5g
- Net Carbs: 7g
- Protein: 13g
- Fat: 14g

These low-carb pancakes are a great option for those with type 1 diabetes, as they are higher in protein and fiber, and lower in carbs compared to traditional pancakes. The fresh fruit adds natural sweetness and nutrients.

5. Berry Smoothie with Protein Powder

Ingredients:

- 1 cup unsweetened almond milk
- 1/2 cup frozen mixed berries
 (such as raspberries, blueberries, strawberries)
- 1 scoop vanilla or unflavored protein powder
- 1 tbsp ground flaxseed
- 1 tsp honey (optional)
- Ice cubes (optional)

Breakfast

PreparationTime: 5 minutes
Total Time: 5 minutes
Serves: 1

↓↓

1. Add the almond milk, frozen berries, protein powder, and ground flaxseed to a high-powered blender.

2. Blend on high speed until the mixture is smooth and creamy, about 1 minute.

3. If a thicker consistency is desired, add a few ice cubes and blend again briefly.

4. Taste and add the honey if a sweeter smoothie is preferred.

5. Pour the smoothie into a glass and enjoy immediately.

Nutrition Information (per serving):
- Calories: 220
- Total Carbs: 16g
- Fiber: 7g
- Net Carbs: 9g
- Protein: 20g
- Fat: 8g

This berry smoothie is a great option for adults with type 1 diabetes as it provides a balance of protein, fiber, and healthy fats to help stabilize blood sugar levels. The berries add natural sweetness and antioxidants, while the protein powder helps build and maintain muscle mass. Be sure to adjust insulin dosage accordingly.

6. Almond Flour Muffins with Blueberries

Ingredients:

- 2 cups almond flour
- 1/4 cup granulated erythritol or other low-carb sweetener
- 1 tsp baking powder
- 1/4 tsp salt
- 3 large eggs
- 1/4 cup unsweetened almond milk
- 2 tbsp melted coconut oil or unsalted butter
- 1 tsp vanilla extract
- 3/4 cup fresh or frozen blueberries

Breakfast

PreparationTime: 10 minutes
Cook Time: 20-22 minutes
Total Time: 30-32 minutes
Serves: 6 muffins

↓↓

1. Preheat the oven to 350°F (175°C). Grease a 6-cup muffin tin or line with paper liners.

2. In a medium bowl, whisk together the almond flour, erythritol, baking powder, and salt.

3. In a separate bowl, beat the eggs. Then stir in the almond milk, melted coconut oil, and vanilla extract.

4. Pour the wet ingredients into the dry ingredients and mix until just combined. Gently fold in the blueberries.

5. Divide the batter evenly among the prepared muffin cups, filling them about 3/4 full.

6. Bake for 20-22 minutes, or until a toothpick inserted into the center comes out clean.

7. Allow the muffins to cool in the tin for 5 minutes before transferring to a wire rack to cool completely.

Nutrition Information (per muffin):
- Calories: 200
- Total Carbs: 8g
- Fiber: 3g
- Net Carbs: 5g
- Protein: 7g
- Fat: 17g

These almond flour muffins are a great option for adults with type 1 diabetes as they are low in net carbs, high in healthy fats, and provide a good amount of protein. The blueberries add natural sweetness and antioxidants. Be sure to adjust insulin dosage accordingly.

7. Scrambled Eggs with Vegetables

Ingredients:

- 3 large eggs
- 1 tbsp olive oil
- 1/4 cup diced bell pepper
- 1/4 cup diced onion
- 1 cup spinach, chopped
- 2 tbsp shredded cheddar cheese (optional)
- Salt and pepper to taste

Breakfast

PreparationTime: 10 minutes
Cook Time: 10 minutes
Total Time: 20 minutes
Serves: 1

↓↓

1. In a small bowl, beat the eggs lightly with a fork until well combined.

2. Heat the olive oil in a non-stick skillet over medium heat.

3. Add the diced bell pepper and onion to the skillet. Sauté for 2-3 minutes, until the vegetables start to soften.

4. Pour the beaten eggs into the skillet and let them sit for 20-30 seconds to set the bottom.

5. Use a spatula to gently push the cooked egg towards the center, tilting the pan to allow the uncooked egg to flow to the edges.

6. When the eggs are mostly set but still a bit runny on top, stir in the chopped spinach.

7. Continue cooking, stirring occasionally, until the eggs are fully cooked through, about 2-3 minutes.

8. Remove from heat and season with salt and pepper to taste. If desired, sprinkle the shredded cheddar cheese over the top. Serve the scrambled eggs with vegetables immediately.

Nutrition Information (per serving):
- Calories: 280
- Total Carbs: 8g
- Fiber: 2g
- Net Carbs: 6g
- Protein: 20g
- Fat: 19g

This scrambled egg dish is a great option for adults with type 1 diabetes as it is high in protein, moderate in carbs, and provides a variety of nutrient-dense vegetables. The healthy fats from the olive oil and optional cheese can help stabilize blood sugar levels. Be sure to adjust insulin dosage accordingly.

8. Overnight Oats with Flaxseed and Nuts

Ingredients:

Breakfast

- 1/2 cup old-fashioned rolled oats
- 1/4 cup unsweetened almond milk
- 1 tbsp chia seeds
- 1 tbsp ground flaxseed
- 1 tbsp chopped walnuts or almonds
- 1 tsp cinnamon
- 1 tsp vanilla extract
- 1-2 tsp low-carb sweetener (such as erythritol or stevia), optional

PreparationTime: 5 minutes
Chilling Time: 8 hours or overnight
Total Time: 8 hours 5 minutes
Serves: 1

↓↓

1. In a medium-sized jar or container with a lid, combine the rolled oats, almond milk, chia seeds, ground flaxseed, chopped nuts, cinnamon, and vanilla extract.

2. If desired, stir in 1-2 tsp of a low-carb sweetener to taste.

3. Secure the lid and refrigerate the overnight oats for at least 8 hours or overnight.

4. When ready to serve, give the mixture a good stir. You may need to add a splash of extra almond milk if it has thickened too much.

5. Enjoy the overnight oats chilled, either as-is or with additional toppings like fresh berries, if desired.

Nutrition Information (per serving):
- Calories: 280
- Total Carbs: 25g
- Fiber: 8g
- Net Carbs: 17g
- Protein: 10g
- Fat: 15g

This overnight oats recipe is a great option for adults with type 1 diabetes. The combination of fiber-rich oats, healthy fats from the nuts and flaxseed, and moderate carbs can help stabilize blood sugar levels. Be sure to adjust insulin dosage accordingly.

9. Quinoa Breakfast Bowl with Apples and Cinnamon

Ingredients:

- 1/2 cup cooked quinoa, cooled
- 1/2 cup unsweetened almond milk
- 1 small apple, diced
- 1 tbsp chopped walnuts
- 1 tsp ground cinnamon
- 1 tsp vanilla extract
- 1 tsp honey (optional)

Breakfast

PreparationTime: 10 minutes
Cook Time: 15 minutes
Total Time: 25 minutes
Serves: 1

↓↓

1. In a medium bowl, combine the cooked quinoa and almond milk. Stir to mix well.

2. Add the diced apple, chopped walnuts, cinnamon, and vanilla extract. Stir to combine.

3. If desired, drizzle the honey over the top and stir again.

4. Serve the quinoa breakfast bowl warm or chilled, as preferred.

Nutrition Information (per serving):
- Calories: 300
- Total Carbs: 40g
- Fiber: 7g
- Net Carbs: 33g
- Protein: 8g
- Fat: 12g

This quinoa breakfast bowl is a great option for adults with type 1 diabetes. Quinoa is a whole grain that is high in fiber and protein, which can help regulate blood sugar levels. The apples provide natural sweetness, while the cinnamon and walnuts add flavor and healthy fats.

Be sure to adjust your insulin dosage accordingly, as the carb content in this dish is moderate. You can also adjust the amount of honey or sweetener used to suit your personal preferences and blood sugar needs.

10. Egg White and Veggie Frittata

Ingredients:

Breakfast

- 8 large egg whites
- 1/4 cup unsweetened almond milk
- 1/4 tsp salt
- 1/4 tsp black pepper
- 1 tbsp olive oil
- 1 cup diced bell peppers
- 1/2 cup diced onions
- 1 cup chopped spinach
- 2 tbsp crumbled feta cheese (optional)

PreparationTime: 10 minutes
Cook Time: 20 minutes
Total Time: 30 minutes
Serves: 4

↓↓↓

1. Preheat your oven to 375°F (190°C).

2. In a medium bowl, whisk together the egg whites, almond milk, salt, and black pepper until well combined.

3. Heat the olive oil in a 9-inch oven-safe non-stick skillet over medium heat.

4. Add the diced bell peppers and onions to the skillet. Sauté for 3-4 minutes, until the vegetables start to soften.

5. Add the chopped spinach to the skillet and cook for an additional 1-2 minutes, until the spinach is wilted.

6. Pour the egg white mixture over the vegetables in the skillet. Gently stir to distribute the vegetables evenly.

7. If using, sprinkle the crumbled feta cheese over the top of the frittata.

8. Transfer the skillet to the preheated oven and bake for 15-20 minutes, or until the frittata is set and lightly golden on top.

9. Remove the frittata from the oven and let it cool for 5 minutes before slicing and serving.

Nutrition Information (per serving):
- Calories: 120 - Total Carbs: 6g - Fiber: 2g - Net Carbs: 4g - Protein: 15g - Fat: 5g

This egg white and veggie frittata is a great option for adults with type 1 diabetes. It's high in protein, low in carbs, and packed with nutrient-dense vegetables. The healthy fats from the olive oil and optional feta cheese can help stabilize blood sugar levels. Be sure to adjust insulin dosage accordingly.

11. Chia Seed Pudding with Almond Milk

Ingredients:

- 1/4 cup chia seeds
- 1 cup unsweetened almond milk
- 1 tsp vanilla extract
- 1/2 tsp ground cinnamon
- 1-2 tsp low-carb sweetener (such as erythritol or stevia), optional

Toppings (optional):
- Fresh berries
- Chopped nuts (such as almonds or walnuts)
- Unsweetened shredded coconut

Breakfast

PreparationTime: 5 minutes
Chilling Time: 2-4 hours
Total Time: 2-4 hours 5 minutes
Serves: 2

↓↓↓

1. In a medium bowl or mason jar, combine the chia seeds, almond milk, vanilla extract, and cinnamon. Stir well to mix.

2. If desired, add 1-2 tsp of a low-carb sweetener and stir again to incorporate.

3. Cover the bowl or seal the jar and refrigerate for 2-4 hours, or until the chia seeds have thickened the mixture into a pudding-like consistency. Stir occasionally during this time.

4. Once the chia seed pudding has set, divide it into two serving bowls or glasses.

5. Top the pudding with your desired toppings, such as fresh berries, chopped nuts, and/or unsweetened shredded coconut.

6. Serve chilled and enjoy!

Nutrition Information (per serving):
- Calories: 160 - Total Carbs: 12g
- Fiber: 8g - Net Carbs: 4g
- Protein: 5g - Fat: 10g

This chia seed pudding is a great option for adults with type 1 diabetes. The chia seeds provide fiber, protein, and healthy fats to help stabilize blood sugar levels. The unsweetened almond milk and optional low-carb sweetener keep the carb count low. Adjust the sweetener to your personal taste preferences and blood sugar needs.

12. Cottage Cheese with Sliced Peaches

Ingredients: **Breakfast**

- 1/2 cup low-fat cottage cheese   **PreparationTime: 5 minutes**
- 1/2 medium peach, sliced   **Total Time: 5 minutes**
- 1 tsp honey (optional)   **Serves: 1**
- Cinnamon (optional)

↓↓↓

1. Scoop the cottage cheese into a small bowl or serving dish.

2. Arrange the sliced peach on top of the cottage cheese.

3. If desired, drizzle the honey over the top of the peaches.

4. Sprinkle a light dusting of cinnamon over the dish, if desired.

Nutrition Information (per serving):
- Calories: 150
- Total Carbs: 12g
- Fiber: 2g
- Net Carbs: 10g
- Protein: 15g
- Fat: 3g

This cottage cheese and peach dish is a great option for adults with type 1 diabetes. The cottage cheese provides a good source of protein, while the peaches add natural sweetness and fiber. The honey is optional, as the peaches provide enough natural sweetness on their own.

The combination of protein, fiber, and moderate carbs from the peaches can help stabilize blood sugar levels. Be sure to adjust your insulin dosage accordingly.

You can also try this with other fresh fruit, such as berries or sliced apples, if you prefer. Just be mindful of the carb content of the fruit.

13. Whole Grain Toast with Avocado and Tomato

Ingredients:

- 2 slices whole grain or sprouted bread
- 1/2 medium avocado, mashed
- 1 medium tomato, sliced
- 1 tbsp olive oil
- Salt and pepper to taste

Breakfast

PreparationTime: 5 minutes
Total Time: 5 minutes
Serves: 1

↓↓↓

1. Toast the two slices of whole grain or sprouted bread until lightly golden.

2. Spread the mashed avocado evenly over the toasted bread slices.

3. Arrange the sliced tomatoes on top of the avocado.

4. Drizzle the olive oil over the tomatoes.

5. Season with a pinch of salt and freshly ground black pepper.

Nutrition Information (per serving):
- Calories: 300
- Total Carbs: 30g
- Fiber: 10g
- Net Carbs: 20g
- Protein: 8g
- Fat: 18g

This whole grain toast with avocado and tomato is a great option for adults with type 1 diabetes. The whole grain bread provides complex carbs and fiber, while the avocado and olive oil offer healthy fats to help stabilize blood sugar levels.

The tomatoes add natural sweetness, vitamins, and antioxidants. Be sure to adjust your insulin dosage accordingly, as the carb content in this dish is moderate.

You can also try adding a sprinkle of feta cheese or a fried egg on top for extra protein if desired.

14. Greek Yogurt Parfait with Nuts and Seeds

Ingredients: **Breakfast**

- 1 cup plain Greek yogurt   **PreparationTime: 5 minutes**
- 2 tbsp mixed nuts (such as almonds, walnuts, pecans)   **Total Time: 5 minutes**
- 1 tbsp mixed seeds (such as chia, flax, pumpkin)   **Serves: 1**
- 1/4 cup fresh berries (such as blueberries, raspberries, strawberries)
- 1 tsp honey (optional)

↓↓

1. In a parfait glass or bowl, layer half of the Greek yogurt.

2. Sprinkle half of the mixed nuts and seeds over the yogurt.

3. Top with half of the fresh berries.

4. Repeat the layers, ending with the remaining yogurt, nuts, seeds, and berries.

5. If desired, drizzle the honey over the top of the parfait.

Nutrition Information (per serving):
- Calories: 280
- Total Carbs: 18g
- Fiber: 6g
- Net Carbs: 12g
- Protein: 20g
- Fat: 15g

This Greek yogurt parfait is a great option for adults with type 1 diabetes. The Greek yogurt provides a good source of protein, while the nuts and seeds offer healthy fats and fiber to help stabilize blood sugar levels.

The fresh berries add natural sweetness and antioxidants. The honey is optional, as the berries provide enough natural sweetness on their own.

Be sure to adjust your insulin dosage accordingly, as the carb content in this dish is moderate.

15. Breakfast Burrito with Black Beans and Veggies

Ingredients:

- 1 whole wheat tortilla or low-carb wrap
- 1/2 cup cooked black beans, rinsed and drained
- 2 large eggs, scrambled
- 1/4 cup diced bell pepper
- 1/4 cup diced onion
- 1 cup spinach, chopped
- 2 tbsp shredded cheddar cheese (optional)
- 1 tbsp salsa (optional)
- Salt and pepper to taste

Breakfast

PreparationTime: 10 minutes
Cook Time: 10 minutes
Total Time: 20 minutes
Serves: 1

↓↓

1. In a non-stick skillet, sauté the diced bell pepper and onion over medium heat for 2-3 minutes until softened.

2. Add the scrambled eggs to the skillet and cook, stirring occasionally, until the eggs are fully cooked.

3. Stir in the black beans and chopped spinach. Cook for an additional 1-2 minutes until the spinach is wilted.

4. Season the egg and vegetable mixture with salt and pepper to taste.

5. Lay the whole wheat tortilla or low-carb wrap on a flat surface. Spoon the egg and vegetable mixture onto the center of the tortilla.

6. If using, sprinkle the shredded cheddar cheese over the top.

7. Fold the bottom of the tortilla up, then fold in the sides and roll up tightly to create a burrito.

8. Serve the breakfast burrito warm, with salsa on the side if desired.

Nutrition Information (per serving):
- Calories: 350 - Total Carbs: 35g
- Fiber: 9g - Net Carbs: 26g
- Protein: 22g - Fat: 15g

This breakfast burrito is a great option for adults with type 1 diabetes. The combination of high-fiber black beans, scrambled eggs, and sautéed vegetables provides a balanced meal with a moderate amount of carbs. The whole wheat tortilla or low-carb wrap helps keep the overall carb content in check. Be sure to adjust your insulin dosage accordingly.

16. Baked Egg Cups with Spinach and Cheese

Ingredients:

- 6 large eggs
- 1/2 cup unsweetened almond milk
- 1 cup fresh spinach, chopped
- 1/4 cup shredded cheddar cheese
- 1 tbsp grated Parmesan cheese
- 1/4 tsp salt
- 1/4 tsp black pepper

Breakfast

PreparationTime: 10 minutes
Cook Time: 20 minutes
Total Time: 30 minutes
Serves: 6 egg cups

↓↓↓

1. Preheat your oven to 350°F (175°C). Grease a 6-cup muffin tin with non-stick cooking spray.

2. In a medium bowl, whisk together the eggs and almond milk until well combined.

3. Stir in the chopped spinach, shredded cheddar cheese, Parmesan cheese, salt, and black pepper.

4. Divide the egg mixture evenly among the prepared muffin cups, filling them about 3/4 full.

5. Bake for 18-20 minutes, or until the egg cups are set and lightly golden on top.

6. Remove the muffin tin from the oven and let the egg cups cool for 5 minutes before gently removing them from the tin.

7. Serve the baked egg cups warm, either on their own or with a side of roasted vegetables or a small salad.

Nutrition Information (per serving):
- Calories: 110 - Total Carbs: 2g - Fiber: 1g - Net Carbs: 1g - Protein: 10g - Fat: 7g

These baked egg cups are a great option for adults with type 1 diabetes. They are low in carbs, high in protein, and packed with nutrient-dense spinach. The combination of eggs, cheese, and healthy fats can help stabilize blood sugar levels.

Be sure to adjust your insulin dosage accordingly, as the carb content in this dish is very low. You can also experiment with different vegetable or cheese combinations to suit your preferences.

17. Protein-Packed Smoothie with Spinach and Almond Milk

Ingredients:

- 1 cup unsweetened almond milk
- 1 scoop vanilla or unflavored protein powder
- 1 cup fresh spinach
- 1/2 cup frozen berries (such as blueberries, raspberries, or strawberries)
- 1 tbsp ground flaxseed
- 1 tsp honey (optional)
- Ice cubes (optional)

Breakfast

PreparationTime: 5 minutes
Total Time: 5 minutes
Serves: 1

↓↓

1. Add the almond milk, protein powder, spinach, frozen berries, and ground flaxseed to a high-powered blender.

2. Blend on high speed until the mixture is smooth and creamy, about 1 minute.

3. If a thicker consistency is desired, add a few ice cubes and blend again briefly.

4. Taste the smoothie and add the honey if a sweeter flavor is preferred.

5. Pour the smoothie into a glass and enjoy immediately.

Nutrition Information (per serving):
- Calories: 270
- Total Carbs: 20g
- Fiber: 7g
- Net Carbs: 13g
- Protein: 24g
- Fat: 10g

This protein-packed smoothie is an excellent choice for adults with type 1 diabetes. The combination of protein-rich powder, fiber-filled spinach, and healthy fats from the flaxseed can help stabilize blood sugar levels.

The berries provide natural sweetness and antioxidants, while the optional honey allows you to adjust the sweetness to your taste preferences and blood sugar needs.

Be sure to adjust your insulin dosage accordingly, as the carb content in this smoothie is moderate.

18. Low-Carb Breakfast Casserole

Ingredients:

Breakfast

- 8 large eggs
- 1/2 cup unsweetened almond milk
- 1 cup diced bell peppers
- 1 cup diced onions
- 1 cup chopped spinach
- 1/2 cup shredded cheddar cheese
- 1/4 cup crumbled feta cheese
- 1 tsp dried oregano
- 1/2 tsp salt
- 1/4 tsp black pepper

PreparationTime: 15 minutes
Cook Time: 35-40 minutes
Total Time: 50-55 minutes
Serves: 6

↓↓

1. Preheat your oven to 375°F (190°C). Grease a 9x13 inch baking dish with non-stick cooking spray.

2. In a large bowl, whisk together the eggs and almond milk until well combined.

3. Stir in the diced bell peppers, onions, chopped spinach, shredded cheddar cheese, crumbled feta cheese, dried oregano, salt, and black pepper.

4. Pour the egg mixture into the prepared baking dish, spreading it out evenly.

5. Bake for 35-40 minutes, or until the casserole is set and the top is lightly golden.

6. Remove the casserole from the oven and let it cool for 5-10 minutes before slicing and serving.

Nutrition Information (per serving:
- Calories: 180 - Total Carbs: 6g - Fiber: 2g - Net Carbs: 4g - Protein: 16g - Fat: 12g

This low-carb breakfast casserole is an excellent option for adults with type 1 diabetes. It's high in protein, moderate in carbs, and packed with nutrient-dense vegetables. The combination of eggs, cheese, and healthy fats can help stabilize blood sugar levels.

Be sure to adjust your insulin dosage accordingly, as the carb content in this dish is relatively low. You can also experiment with different vegetable or cheese combinations to suit your preferences.

19. Whole Wheat English Muffin with Peanut Butter

Ingredients:

- 1 whole wheat English muffin
- 2 tbsp natural peanut butter (no added sugar)
- 1 tsp chia seeds (optional)

Breakfast

PreparationTime: 5 minutes
Total Time: 5 minutes
Serves: 1

↓↓

1. Toast the whole wheat English muffin until lightly golden.

2. Spread the natural peanut butter evenly over the toasted muffin.

3. If desired, sprinkle the chia seeds over the peanut butter.

Nutrition Information (per serving):
- Calories: 280
- Total Carbs: 28g
- Fiber: 6g
- Net Carbs: 22g
- Protein: 12g
- Fat: 14g

This whole wheat English muffin with peanut butter is a great option for adults with type 1 diabetes. The whole grain muffin provides complex carbs and fiber, while the peanut butter offers a source of protein and healthy fats.

The combination of carbs, protein, and healthy fats can help stabilize blood sugar levels. Be sure to choose a natural peanut butter without added sugars.

You can also add the optional chia seeds to boost the fiber and nutrient content of the dish.

Remember to adjust your insulin dosage accordingly, as the carb content in this meal is moderate.

20. Fruit and Nut Breakfast Bars

Ingredients:

Breakfast

Preparation Time: 15 minutes
Cook Time: 25 minutes
Total Time: 40 minutes
Serves: 8 bars

- 1 cup almond flour
- 1/4 cup coconut flour
- 1/4 cup ground flaxseed
- 1 tsp baking powder
- 1/4 tsp salt
- 2 large eggs
- 1/4 cup unsweetened almond milk
- 2 tbsp coconut oil, melted
- 1 tsp vanilla extract
- 1/2 cup chopped mixed nuts (such as almonds, walnuts, pecans)
- 1/2 cup diced dried fruit (such as apricots, cranberries, or cherries)

↓↓

1. Preheat your oven to 350°F (175°C). Line an 8x8 inch baking pan with parchment paper.

2. In a medium bowl, whisk together the almond flour, coconut flour, ground flaxseed, baking powder, and salt.

3. In a separate bowl, beat the eggs. Then stir in the almond milk, melted coconut oil, and vanilla extract.

4. Pour the wet ingredients into the dry ingredients and mix until just combined. Fold in the chopped nuts and diced dried fruit.

5. Spread the batter evenly into the prepared baking pan.

6. Bake for 25-30 minutes, or until the bars are lightly golden and a toothpick inserted in the center comes out clean. Allow the bars to cool completely in the pan before cutting into 8 equal pieces.

Nutrition Information (per serving):
- Calories: 220 - Total Carbs: 14g - Fiber: 5g - Net Carbs: 9g - Protein: 7g - Fat: 16g

These fruit and nut breakfast bars are a great option for adults with type 1 diabetes. The combination of almond and coconut flours, along with the healthy fats from the nuts and coconut oil, helps keep the carb content moderate while providing a good source of protein and fiber. The dried fruit adds natural sweetness, while the nuts provide crunch and additional nutrients. Be sure to adjust your insulin dosage accordingly, as the carb content in these bars is still moderate.

1. Grilled Chicken Salad with Mixed Greens

Ingredients:

- 4 oz grilled chicken breast, sliced
- 2 cups mixed greens (such as spinach, arugula, kale)
- 1/2 cup cherry tomatoes, halved
- 1/4 cup cucumber, sliced
- 2 tbsp crumbled feta cheese
- 1 tbsp olive oil
- 1 tbsp balsamic vinegar
- Salt and pepper to taste

Lunch

PreparationTime: 10 minutes
Cook Time: 10-12 minutes
Total Time: 20-22 minutes
Serves: 1

↓↓

1. Preheat your grill or grill pan to medium-high heat. Season the chicken breast with a pinch of salt and pepper.

2. Grill the chicken for 5-6 minutes per side, or until it reaches an internal temperature of 165°F (75°C). Remove from heat and let rest for a few minutes, then slice the chicken.

3. In a large salad bowl, combine the mixed greens, cherry tomatoes, cucumber, and crumbled feta cheese.

4. Drizzle the olive oil and balsamic vinegar over the salad and toss gently to coat.

5. Top the salad with the grilled chicken slices.

6. Season with additional salt and pepper to taste.

Nutrition Information (per serving):
- Calories: 320 - Total Carbs: 10g - Fiber: 3g - Net Carbs: 7g - Protein: 35g - Fat: 16g

This grilled chicken salad is an excellent option for adults with type 1 diabetes. The combination of lean protein from the chicken, healthy fats from the olive oil and feta, and fiber-rich greens can help stabilize blood sugar levels.

The net carb content is relatively low, making it a great choice for those managing their diabetes. Be sure to adjust your insulin dosage accordingly.

You can also experiment with different vegetable toppings or swap the balsamic vinegar for a low-carb dressing of your choice.

2. Quinoa and Black Bean Salad

Ingredients:

- 1 cup cooked quinoa, cooled
- 1 (15 oz) can black beans, rinsed and drained
- 1 cup diced bell peppers (mix of red, yellow, and/or orange)
- 1/2 cup diced red onion
- 1/2 cup diced cucumber
- 1/4 cup chopped fresh cilantro
- 2 tbsp olive oil
- 2 tbsp lime juice
- 1 tsp ground cumin
- 1/4 tsp salt
- 1/4 tsp black pepper

Lunch

PreparationTime: 15 minutes
Cook Time: 15 minutes
Total Time: 30 minutes
Serves: 4

↓↓

1. In a large bowl, combine the cooked quinoa, black beans, diced bell peppers, red onion, cucumber, and chopped cilantro.

2. In a small bowl, whisk together the olive oil, lime juice, cumin, salt, and black pepper.

3. Pour the dressing over the quinoa and bean mixture and toss gently to coat.

4. Refrigerate the salad for at least 15 minutes to allow the flavors to meld.

5. Serve chilled or at room temperature.

Nutrition Information (per serving):
- Calories: 220 - Total Carbs: 28g - Fiber: 7g - Net Carbs: 21g - Protein: 8g - Fat: 9g

This quinoa and black bean salad is a great option for adults with type 1 diabetes. The combination of high-fiber quinoa, protein-rich black beans, and nutrient-dense vegetables provides a balanced and satisfying meal.

The healthy fats from the olive oil and the fiber from the beans and quinoa can help regulate blood sugar levels. Be sure to adjust your insulin dosage accordingly, as the carb content in this dish is moderate.

You can also customize the salad by adding other vegetables, herbs, or a sprinkle of feta cheese to suit your preferences.

3. Turkey and Avocado Lettuce Wraps

Ingredients:

- 4 oz sliced turkey breast
- 1/2 medium avocado, sliced
- 2 tbsp plain Greek yogurt
- 1 tsp Dijon mustard
- 1/4 tsp dried dill
- Salt and pepper to taste
- 4 large lettuce leaves (such as romaine or butter lettuce)

Lunch

PreparationTime: 10 minutes
Total Time: 10 minutes
Serves: 2

↓↓

1. In a small bowl, mix together the Greek yogurt, Dijon mustard, and dried dill. Season with a pinch of salt and pepper.

2. Lay the lettuce leaves flat on a clean surface.

3. Divide the sliced turkey and avocado evenly among the lettuce leaves.

4. Drizzle the yogurt-mustard dressing over the turkey and avocado.

5. Carefully wrap the lettuce around the fillings to create the lettuce wraps.

6. Serve immediately.

Nutrition Information (per serving):
- Calories: 180 - Total Carbs: 6g - Fiber: 4g - Net Carbs: 2g - Protein: 18g - Fat: 10g

These turkey and avocado lettuce wraps are an excellent option for adults with type 1 diabetes. The combination of lean protein from the turkey, healthy fats from the avocado, and low-carb lettuce leaves makes for a balanced and blood sugar-friendly meal.

The Greek yogurt-based dressing adds a creamy texture and a touch of flavor without significantly increasing the carb content.

Be sure to adjust your insulin dosage accordingly, as the net carb content in this dish is very low.

You can also experiment with different protein sources, such as grilled chicken or tuna, or add extra vegetables to the wraps.

4. Greek Salad with Chicken

Ingredients:

Lunch

- 4 oz grilled or baked chicken breast, sliced
- 2 cups chopped romaine lettuce
- 1/2 cup diced cucumber
- 1/4 cup diced tomatoes
- 2 tbsp crumbled feta cheese
- 2 tbsp sliced kalamata olives
- 1 tbsp olive oil
- 1 tbsp red wine vinegar
- 1 tsp dried oregano
- 1/4 tsp salt
- 1/4 tsp black pepper

PreparationTime: 15 minutes
Cook Time: 10 minutes
Total Time: 25 minutes
Serves: 2

↓↓

1. In a large salad bowl, combine the chopped romaine lettuce, diced cucumber, diced tomatoes, crumbled feta cheese, and sliced kalamata olives.

2. In a small bowl, whisk together the olive oil, red wine vinegar, dried oregano, salt, and black pepper to make the dressing.

3. Add the sliced grilled or baked chicken to the salad.

4. Drizzle the dressing over the salad and toss gently to coat.

Nutrition Information (per serving):
- Calories: 280 - Total Carbs: 10g - Fiber: 3g - Net Carbs: 7g - Protein: 30g - Fat: 14g

This Greek salad with chicken is an excellent option for adults with type 1 diabetes. The combination of lean protein from the chicken, healthy fats from the olive oil and feta, and fiber-rich vegetables can help stabilize blood sugar levels.

The net carb content is relatively low, making it a great choice for those managing their diabetes. Be sure to adjust your insulin dosage accordingly.

You can also experiment with different vegetable toppings or swap the red wine vinegar for a low-carb dressing of your choice.

5. Vegetable and Lentil Soup

Ingredients:

Lunch

- 1 tbsp olive oil
- 1 onion, diced
- 2 carrots, peeled and diced
- 2 celery stalks, diced
- 3 garlic cloves, minced
- 1 cup dried brown or green lentils, rinsed
- 4 cups low-sodium vegetable broth
- 1 (14.5 oz) can diced tomatoes
- 2 cups chopped kale or spinach
- 1 tsp dried thyme
- 1/2 tsp dried oregano
- Salt and pepper to taste

PreparationTime: 15 minutes
Cook Time: 30 minutes
Total Time: 45 minutes
Serves: 4

↓↓

1. In a large pot or Dutch oven, heat the olive oil over medium heat.

2. Add the diced onion, carrots, and celery. Sauté for 5-7 minutes, until the vegetables start to soften.

3. Stir in the minced garlic and cook for an additional minute.

4. Add the rinsed lentils, vegetable broth, diced tomatoes, chopped kale or spinach, dried thyme, and dried oregano.

5. Bring the soup to a boil, then reduce the heat and let it simmer for 25-30 minutes, or until the lentils are tender.

6. Season the soup with salt and pepper to taste. Serve the vegetable and lentil soup hot.

Nutrition Information (per serving):
- Calories: 250 - Total Carbs: 35g - Fiber: 12g - Net Carbs: 23g - Protein: 13g - Fat: 6g

This vegetable and lentil soup is a great option for adults with type 1 diabetes. The combination of high-fiber lentils, nutrient-dense vegetables, and low-sodium broth provides a balanced and satisfying meal.

The fiber and protein from the lentils can help regulate blood sugar levels. Be sure to adjust your insulin dosage accordingly, as the carb content in this dish is moderate.

You can also customize the soup by adding other vegetables, herbs, or a sprinkle of grated Parmesan cheese to suit your preferences.

6. Spinach and Chickpea Salad

Ingredients:

Lunch

- 5 oz baby spinach leaves
- 1 (15 oz) can chickpeas, drained and rinsed
- 1 cup cherry tomatoes, halved
- 1/2 red onion, thinly sliced
- 1/4 cup crumbled feta cheese
- 2 tbsp olive oil
- 2 tbsp red wine vinegar
- 1 tsp Dijon mustard
- 1 tsp honey
- 1/4 tsp salt
- 1/4 tsp black pepper

PreparationTime: 15 minutes
Total Time: 15 minutes
Serves: 4

↓↓

1. In a large salad bowl, combine the baby spinach, chickpeas, cherry tomatoes, and red onion.

2. In a small bowl, whisk together the olive oil, red wine vinegar, Dijon mustard, honey, salt, and black pepper to make the dressing.

3. Pour the dressing over the salad and toss gently to coat.

4. Sprinkle the crumbled feta cheese over the top.

5. Serve immediately. Enjoy!

This salad is packed with protein from the chickpeas, vitamins and minerals from the spinach, and a tangy, flavorful dressing. It makes a great light lunch or side dish.

7. Stuffed Bell Peppers with Ground Turkey

Ingredients:

- 6 bell peppers (any color)
- 1 lb ground turkey
- 1 cup cooked rice
- 1 small onion, diced
- 2 cloves garlic, minced
- 1 tsp dried oregano
- 1 tsp dried basil
- 1/2 tsp salt
- 1/4 tsp black pepper
- 1 cup shredded mozzarella cheese

Lunch

PreparationTime: 15 minutes
Cook Time: 40 minutes
Total Time: 55 minutes
Serves: 6

↓↓↓

1. Preheat oven to 375°F.

2. Cut the tops off the bell peppers and remove the seeds and membranes. Place the peppers in a baking dish.

3. In a skillet over medium heat, cook the ground turkey, onion, and garlic until the turkey is browned and the onion is softened, about 5-7 minutes. Drain any excess fat.

4. Stir in the cooked rice, oregano, basil, salt, and pepper.

5. Stuff each bell pepper cavity with the turkey and rice mixture, packing it in tightly.

6. Top each stuffed pepper with shredded mozzarella cheese.

7. Cover the baking dish with foil and bake for 30 minutes.

8. Remove the foil and bake for an additional 10-15 minutes, until the peppers are tender and the cheese is melted and bubbly.

9. Serve hot. Enjoy!

8. Tuna Salad with Mixed Vegetables

Ingredients:

Lunch

- 2 (5 oz) cans tuna, drained
- 1/2 cup diced cucumber
- 1/2 cup diced bell pepper
- 1/2 cup diced celery
- 1/4 cup diced red onion
- 2 tbsp plain Greek yogurt
- 1 tbsp Dijon mustard
- 1 tbsp lemon juice
- 1/4 tsp salt
- 1/4 tsp black pepper
- 2 cups mixed greens (such as spinach, arugula, or kale)

PreparationTime: 15 minutes
Total Time: 15 minutes
Serves: 4

↓↓

1. In a medium bowl, combine the drained tuna, diced cucumber, bell pepper, celery, and red onion.

2. In a small bowl, whisk together the Greek yogurt, Dijon mustard, lemon juice, salt, and black pepper to make the dressing.

3. Pour the dressing over the tuna and vegetable mixture and stir gently to coat.

4. Divide the mixed greens onto 4 plates or bowls.

5. Top the greens with the tuna salad mixture.

6. Serve immediately.

This tuna salad is a great option for adults with type 1 diabetes as it is high in protein from the tuna, low in carbs, and contains a variety of nutrient-dense vegetables. The Greek yogurt in the dressing provides a creamy texture without adding too many carbs. Be sure to adjust portion sizes as needed to fit your individual carb and calorie needs.

9. Chicken and Vegetable Stir-Fry

Ingredients:

Lunch

- 1 lb boneless, skinless chicken breasts,
cut into 1-inch pieces
- 2 tbsp low-sodium soy sauce
- 1 tbsp rice vinegar
- 1 tsp sesame oil
- 1 tsp cornstarch
- 2 tbsp olive oil
- 3 cloves garlic, minced
- 1 tbsp grated fresh ginger
- 1 red bell pepper, sliced
- 1 cup broccoli florets
- 1 cup snow peas
- 1 cup sliced mushrooms
- 2 green onions, sliced
- 1/4 cup low-sodium chicken broth
- Salt and black pepper to taste
- Cooked brown rice, for serving

PreparationTime: 20 minutes
Cook Time: 15 minutes
Total Time: 35 minutes
Serves: 4

↓↓↓

1. In a medium bowl, combine the chicken, soy sauce, rice vinegar, sesame oil, and cornstarch. Toss to coat the chicken and set aside.

2. Heat the olive oil in a large skillet or wok over high heat. Add the garlic and ginger and cook for 1 minute, stirring constantly.

3. Add the chicken mixture and cook for 3-4 minutes, stirring frequently, until the chicken is lightly browned.

4. Add the bell pepper, broccoli, snow peas, and mushrooms. Cook for 5-7 minutes, stirring frequently, until the vegetables are tender-crisp.

5. Pour in the chicken broth and cook for 2-3 minutes, until the sauce has thickened slightly.

6. Remove from heat and stir in the green onions. Season with salt and black pepper to taste.

7. Serve the stir-fry immediately over cooked brown rice.

This chicken and vegetable stir-fry is a quick and healthy meal that is packed with protein, fiber, and nutrients. The combination of lean chicken, fresh vegetables, and a flavorful sauce makes it a great option for a balanced dinner.

10. Whole Grain Wrap with Hummus and Veggies

Ingredients:

Lunch

- 1 (8-inch) whole grain tortilla or wrap
- 2 tbsp hummus
- 1/2 cup sliced cucumber
- 1/4 cup shredded carrots
- 1/4 cup sliced bell pepper
- 2 tbsp crumbled feta cheese
- 1 tbsp chopped fresh parsley (optional)

PreparationTime: 10 minutes
Total Time: 10 minutes
Serves: 1

↓↓

1. Spread the hummus evenly over the whole grain tortilla or wrap.

2. Layer the sliced cucumber, shredded carrots, and sliced bell pepper on top of the hummus.

3. Sprinkle the crumbled feta cheese over the vegetables.

4. If desired, top with chopped fresh parsley.

5. Carefully roll up the wrap, tucking in the sides as you go.

6. Slice the wrap in half diagonally and serve immediately.

This whole grain wrap is a great option for adults with type 1 diabetes as it provides a balance of complex carbohydrates, protein, and healthy fats. The hummus and vegetables add fiber, vitamins, and minerals, while the whole grain wrap helps to control blood sugar levels. The feta cheese provides a boost of protein.

Be sure to adjust the portion size as needed to fit your individual carb and calorie requirements. You can also customize the vegetables used to your personal preferences.

11. Cabbage and Ground Beef Skillet

Ingredients:

- 1 lb lean ground beef
- 1 medium head of cabbage, shredded (about 6 cups)
- 1 medium onion, diced
- 2 cloves garlic, minced
- 1 tsp dried oregano
- 1 tsp paprika
- 1/2 tsp salt
- 1/4 tsp black pepper
- 1/4 cup low-sodium beef or chicken broth
- 2 tbsp apple cider vinegar
- 2 tbsp chopped fresh parsley (optional)

Lunch

PreparationTime: 15 minutes
Cook Time: 20 minutes
Total Time: 35 minutes
Serves: 4

↓↓↓

1. In a large skillet over medium-high heat, cook the ground beef, breaking it up with a wooden spoon, until browned and cooked through, about 5-7 minutes. Drain any excess fat.

2. Add the shredded cabbage, onion, garlic, oregano, paprika, salt, and pepper to the skillet. Stir to combine.

3. Pour in the broth and apple cider vinegar. Bring the mixture to a simmer, then reduce heat to medium-low and cover the skillet.

4. Cook for 15-20 minutes, stirring occasionally, until the cabbage is tender.

5. Remove from heat and stir in the chopped parsley, if using.

6. Serve hot.

This cabbage and ground beef skillet is a great option for adults with type 1 diabetes as it is low in carbs, high in protein, and packed with fiber and nutrients from the cabbage. The apple cider vinegar adds a nice tangy flavor without adding too many carbs.

Be sure to adjust portion sizes as needed to fit your individual carb and calorie requirements. You can also serve this over cauliflower rice or with a side salad for a complete, balanced meal.

13. Shrimp and Avocado Salad

Ingredients:

Lunch

PreparationTime: 15 minutes
Total Time: 15 minutes
Serves: 4

- 1 lb cooked shrimp, peeled and deveined
- 1 avocado, diced
- 1 cup cherry tomatoes, halved
- 1/2 cup diced cucumber
- 1/4 cup diced red onion
- 2 tbsp chopped fresh cilantro
- 2 tbsp lime juice
- 1 tbsp olive oil
- 1/4 tsp salt
- 1/4 tsp black pepper

↓↓

1. In a large bowl, combine the cooked shrimp, diced avocado, cherry tomatoes, diced cucumber, red onion, and chopped cilantro.

2. In a small bowl, whisk together the lime juice, olive oil, salt, and black pepper to make the dressing.

3. Pour the dressing over the shrimp and vegetable mixture and gently toss to coat.

4. Serve immediately or refrigerate until ready to serve.

This shrimp and avocado salad is a great option for adults with type 1 diabetes as it is high in protein, healthy fats, and fiber, while being low in carbs. The combination of shrimp, avocado, and fresh vegetables provides a nutrient-dense and satisfying meal.

The lime juice and olive oil dressing adds a bright, flavorful touch without adding too many carbs. You can adjust the amount of dressing to your preference.

Be sure to adjust portion sizes as needed to fit your individual carb and calorie requirements. You can also serve this salad over a bed of mixed greens for a more substantial meal.

14. Tomato and Mozzarella Caprese Salad

Ingredients:

Lunch
PreparationTime: 10 minutes
Total Time: 10 minutes
Serves: 4

- 1 lb cherry or grape tomatoes, halved
- 8 oz fresh mozzarella cheese, cut into 1-inch cubes
- 1/4 cup fresh basil leaves, chopped
- 2 tbsp balsamic glaze
- 1 tbsp olive oil
- 1/4 tsp salt
- 1/4 tsp black pepper

↓↓

1. In a large bowl, combine the halved tomatoes, mozzarella cheese cubes, and chopped basil leaves.

2. Drizzle the balsamic glaze and olive oil over the salad, then season with salt and black pepper.

3. Gently toss the salad to coat the ingredients with the dressing.

4. Serve immediately or refrigerate until ready to serve.

This Tomato and Mozzarella Caprese Salad is a great option for adults with type 1 diabetes as it is low in carbs, high in protein and healthy fats, and packed with vitamins and antioxidants.

The balsamic glaze provides a sweet and tangy flavor without adding too many carbs. You can adjust the amount of glaze to your preference.

Be sure to choose a high-quality, fresh mozzarella cheese to ensure the best flavor and texture. You can also add a sprinkle of pine nuts or a drizzle of extra-virgin olive oil for additional healthy fats.

Adjust the portion size as needed to fit your individual carb and calorie requirements. This salad can be enjoyed as a light main dish or a side salad.

15. Turkey Chili with Beans

Ingredients:

Lunch

- 1 lb ground turkey
- 1 medium onion, diced
- 3 cloves garlic, minced
- 2 tbsp chili powder
- 1 tsp ground cumin
- 1 tsp dried oregano
- 1/2 tsp smoked paprika
- 1/4 tsp cayenne pepper (optional)
- 1 (15 oz) can diced tomatoes
- 1 (15 oz) can kidney beans, drained and rinsed
- 1 (15 oz) can black beans, drained and rinsed
- 1 cup low-sodium chicken or vegetable broth
- 1/4 tsp salt
- 1/4 tsp black pepper
- Chopped fresh cilantro for garnish (optional)

PreparationTime: 15 minutes
Cook Time: 45 minutes
Total Time: 1 hour
Serves: 6

↓↓

1. In a large pot or Dutch oven over medium-high heat, cook the ground turkey, breaking it up with a wooden spoon, until browned and cooked through, about 5-7 minutes. Drain any excess fat.

2. Add the diced onion and minced garlic to the pot. Cook for 2-3 minutes, stirring frequently, until the onion is translucent.

3. Stir in the chili powder, cumin, oregano, smoked paprika, and cayenne pepper (if using). Cook for 1 minute to toast the spices.

4. Add the diced tomatoes, kidney beans, black beans, and chicken or vegetable broth. Stir to combine.

5. Bring the chili to a simmer, then reduce the heat to medium-low. Simmer for 30-40 minutes, stirring occasionally, until the flavors have melded and the chili has thickened.

6. Season with salt and black pepper to taste. Serve the chili hot, garnished with chopped fresh cilantro if desired.

This turkey chili with beans is a great option for adults with type 1 diabetes as it is high in protein, fiber, and complex carbohydrates, while being relatively low in simple carbs. The combination of lean ground turkey, beans, and spices provides a satisfying and nutrient-dense meal. Be sure to adjust portion sizes as needed to fit your individual carb and calorie requirements. You can also serve the chili over cauliflower rice or with a side salad for a complete, balanced meal.

16. Grilled Salmon with Asparagus

Ingredients:

Lunch

- 4 (6 oz) salmon fillets
- 1 lb asparagus, trimmed
- 2 tbsp olive oil, divided
- 1 tsp lemon zest
- 1 tbsp lemon juice
- 1 tsp Dijon mustard
- 1 clove garlic, minced
- 1/4 tsp salt
- 1/4 tsp black pepper

PreparationTime: 10 minutes
Cook Time: 15 minutes
Total Time: 25 minutes
Serves: 4

↓↓

1. Preheat grill or grill pan to medium-high heat.

2. In a small bowl, whisk together 1 tbsp olive oil, lemon zest, lemon juice, Dijon mustard, garlic, salt, and black pepper to make the dressing.

3. Toss the asparagus with the remaining 1 tbsp olive oil and season with a pinch of salt and pepper.

4. Place the salmon fillets and asparagus on the preheated grill. Cook for 5-7 minutes per side for the salmon, and 8-10 minutes for the asparagus, until both are cooked through.

5. Transfer the grilled salmon and asparagus to a serving platter. Drizzle the lemon-Dijon dressing over the top. Serve immediately.

This grilled salmon and asparagus dish is a great option for adults with type 1 diabetes as it is high in protein, healthy fats, and fiber, while being low in carbs. The lemon-Dijon dressing adds a bright, flavorful touch without adding too many carbs.

Be sure to adjust portion sizes as needed to fit your individual carb and calorie requirements. You can also serve this with a side of roasted or steamed vegetables for a more complete meal.

The salmon and asparagus can be grilled or baked, depending on your preference. Just be sure to adjust the cooking time accordingly.

17. Sweet Potato and Black Bean Bowl

Ingredients:

Lunch

- 2 medium sweet potatoes, peeled and diced
- 1 tbsp olive oil
- 1/2 tsp chili powder
- 1/4 tsp salt
- 1 (15 oz) can black beans, drained and rinsed
- 1 cup cooked quinoa
- 1 cup diced tomatoes
- 1/2 cup diced avocado
- 2 tbsp chopped fresh cilantro
- 1 tbsp lime juice
- 1/4 tsp black pepper

PreparationTime: 15 minutes
Cook Time: 30 minutes
Total Time: 45 minutes
Serves: 4

↓↓↓

1. Preheat the oven to 400°F. Line a baking sheet with parchment paper.

2. In a large bowl, toss the diced sweet potatoes with the olive oil, chili powder, and salt. Spread the sweet potatoes in a single layer on the prepared baking sheet.

3. Roast the sweet potatoes for 25-30 minutes, stirring halfway, until they are tender and lightly browned.

4. In a large bowl, combine the roasted sweet potatoes, drained and rinsed black beans, cooked quinoa, diced tomatoes, diced avocado, chopped cilantro, lime juice, and black pepper. Stir gently to mix.

5. Serve the sweet potato and black bean bowl immediately.

This sweet potato and black bean bowl is a great option for adults with type 1 diabetes as it is high in fiber, complex carbohydrates, protein, and healthy fats, while being relatively low in simple carbs.

The combination of roasted sweet potatoes, black beans, quinoa, and fresh vegetables provides a nutrient-dense and satisfying meal. The lime juice and cilantro add a bright, flavorful touch.

Be sure to adjust portion sizes as needed to fit your individual carb and calorie requirements. You can also customize the ingredients based on your preferences, such as adding different types of beans or vegetables.

18. Chicken Caesar Salad

Ingredients:

- 1 lb boneless, skinless chicken breasts
- 1 tbsp olive oil
- 1/4 tsp salt
- 1/4 tsp black pepper
- 6 cups chopped romaine lettuce
- 1/4 cup grated Parmesan cheese
- 2 tbsp low-fat Caesar dressing
- 2 tbsp chopped fresh parsley (optional)

Lunch

PreparationTime: 15 minutes
Cook Time: 10 minutes
Total Time: 25 minutes
Serves: 4

↓↓

1. Preheat the oven to 400°F. Line a baking sheet with parchment paper.

2. Season the chicken breasts with the salt and black pepper.

3. Heat the olive oil in a large skillet over medium-high heat. Add the chicken and cook for 5-7 minutes per side, until cooked through. Transfer the chicken to the prepared baking sheet.

4. Bake the chicken for an additional 5 minutes to ensure it is fully cooked. Allow to cool slightly, then slice or shred the chicken.

5. In a large salad bowl, combine the chopped romaine lettuce, sliced or shredded chicken, grated Parmesan cheese, and Caesar dressing. Toss gently to coat.

6. Garnish the salad with chopped fresh parsley, if desired. Serve immediately.

This Chicken Caesar Salad is a great option for adults with type 1 diabetes as it is high in protein, low in carbs, and provides a good source of fiber and nutrients from the romaine lettuce.

The low-fat Caesar dressing helps to keep the carb and calorie content in check, while still providing a creamy, flavorful dressing. You can also use a homemade Caesar dressing if preferred.

Be sure to adjust the portion sizes as needed to fit your individual carb and calorie requirements. You can also add additional vegetables, such as cherry tomatoes or cucumber, to increase the fiber and nutrient content.

19. Zucchini Noodles with Marinara Sauce

Ingredients: **Lunch**

- 4 medium zucchini, spiralized or julienned into noodles   **PreparationTime: 15 minutes**
- 1 tbsp olive oil   **Cook Time: 15 minutes**
- 3 cloves garlic, minced   **Total Time: 30 minutes**
- 1 (28 oz) can crushed tomatoes   **Serves: 4**
- 2 tbsp tomato paste
- 1 tsp dried oregano
- 1/2 tsp dried basil
- 1/4 tsp red pepper flakes (optional)
- 1/4 tsp salt
- 1/4 tsp black pepper
- 2 tbsp grated Parmesan cheese (optional)
- Chopped fresh basil for garnish (optional)

↓↓

1. Using a spiralizer or julienne peeler, create zucchini noodles from the 4 medium zucchinis. Set aside.

2. In a large skillet, heat the olive oil over medium heat. Add the minced garlic and cook for 1 minute, stirring constantly, until fragrant.

3. Add the crushed tomatoes, tomato paste, dried oregano, dried basil, red pepper flakes (if using), salt, and black pepper. Stir to combine.

4. Bring the sauce to a simmer and let it cook for 5-7 minutes, stirring occasionally, until slightly thickened.

5. Add the zucchini noodles to the sauce and toss to coat. Cook for an additional 3-5 minutes, until the zucchini noodles are tender but still have a bite.

6. Remove from heat and serve the zucchini noodles with marinara sauce immediately.

7. If desired, top with grated Parmesan cheese and chopped fresh basil.

This zucchini noodle dish is a great option for adults with type 1 diabetes as it is low in carbs, high in fiber, and provides a good source of vitamins and minerals from the zucchini and tomato-based sauce.

The zucchini noodles can be a satisfying and lower-carb alternative to traditional pasta. Be sure to adjust portion sizes as needed to fit your individual carb and calorie requirements.

You can also customize the recipe by adding grilled chicken or sautéed mushrooms for additional protein.

20. Vegetable and Tofu Stir-Fry

Ingredients:

Lunch

PreparationTime: 20 minutes
Cook Time: 15 minutes
Total Time: 35 minutes
Serves: 4

- 1 block (14 oz) extra-firm tofu, drained and cubed
- 2 tbsp low-sodium soy sauce, divided
- 1 tbsp sesame oil
- 1 tbsp rice vinegar
- 1 tsp cornstarch
- 2 tbsp olive oil
- 3 cloves garlic, minced
- 1 tbsp grated fresh ginger
- 1 red bell pepper, sliced
- 1 cup broccoli florets
- 1 cup snow peas
- 1 cup sliced mushrooms
- 2 green onions, sliced
- 1/4 cup low-sodium vegetable broth
- Salt and black pepper to taste
- Cooked cauliflower rice, for serving

↓↓

1. In a medium bowl, combine the cubed tofu, 1 tbsp of the soy sauce, sesame oil, rice vinegar, and cornstarch. Toss to coat the tofu and set aside.

2. Heat the olive oil in a large skillet or wok over high heat. Add the garlic and ginger and cook for 1 minute, stirring constantly.

3. Add the marinated tofu and cook for 3-4 minutes, stirring frequently, until the tofu is lightly browned.

4. Add the sliced bell pepper, broccoli, snow peas, and mushrooms. Cook for 5-7 minutes, stirring frequently, until the vegetables are tender-crisp.

5. Pour in the vegetable broth and remaining 1 tbsp of soy sauce. Cook for 2-3 minutes, until the sauce has thickened slightly.

6. Remove from heat and stir in the sliced green onions. Season with salt and black pepper to taste. Serve the vegetable and tofu stir-fry immediately over cooked cauliflower rice.

This vegetable and tofu stir-fry is a great option for adults with type 1 diabetes as it is high in protein, fiber, and nutrients, while being low in carbs. The combination of tofu, fresh vegetables, and a flavorful sauce makes it a satisfying 𝗍ond balanced meal.

Be sure to adjust portion sizes as needed to fit your individual carb and calorie requirements. You can also customize the vegetables used based on your preferences.

1. Baked Salmon with Lemon and Dill

Ingredients:

- 4 (6 oz) salmon fillets
- 2 tbsp olive oil
- 2 tbsp freshly squeezed lemon juice
- 1 tsp dried dill
- 1/2 tsp garlic powder
- 1/4 tsp salt
- 1/4 tsp black pepper

Dinner

PreparationTime: 10 minutes
Cook Time: 15 minutes
Total Time: 25 minutes
Serves: 4

↓↓↓

1. Preheat the oven to 400°F. Line a baking sheet with parchment paper.

2. In a small bowl, whisk together the olive oil, lemon juice, dried dill, garlic powder, salt, and black pepper to make the marinade.

3. Place the salmon fillets on the prepared baking sheet. Brush the top of each fillet with the lemon-dill marinade, making sure to coat them evenly.

4. Bake the salmon for 12-15 minutes, or until it flakes easily with a fork and reaches an internal temperature of 145°F.

5. Serve the baked salmon immediately, garnished with additional lemon wedges and fresh dill, if desired.

This baked salmon dish is an excellent choice for adults with type 1 diabetes as it is high in protein, healthy fats, and low in carbs. The lemon and dill flavors provide a bright, fresh taste without adding any significant carbohydrates.

To make this meal even more diabetes-friendly, you can serve the salmon with a side of roasted vegetables, such as asparagus or broccoli, or a fresh salad. Adjust the portion size as needed to fit your individual carb and calorie requirements.

The salmon can also be grilled or pan-seared instead of baked, if preferred. Just be sure to adjust the cooking time accordingly.

2. Grilled Chicken with Steamed Broccoli

Ingredients:

- 4 (6 oz) boneless, skinless chicken breasts
- 1 tbsp olive oil
- 1 tsp dried oregano
- 1/2 tsp garlic powder
- 1/4 tsp salt
- 1/4 tsp black pepper
- 1 lb broccoli florets
- 2 tbsp lemon juice
- 1 tbsp chopped fresh parsley (optional)

Dinner

PreparationTime: 10 minutes
Cook Time: 20 minutes
Total Time: 30 minutes
Serves: 4

↓↓↓

1. Preheat grill or grill pan to medium-high heat.

2. In a small bowl, combine the olive oil, dried oregano, garlic powder, salt, and black pepper. Rub the seasoning mixture all over the chicken breasts.

3. Grill the chicken for 6-8 minutes per side, or until it reaches an internal temperature of 165°F.

4. While the chicken is grilling, steam the broccoli florets until tender-crisp, about 5-7 minutes.

5. Transfer the grilled chicken and steamed broccoli to a serving platter. Drizzle the lemon juice over the broccoli and sprinkle with chopped fresh parsley, if desired.

6. Serve immediately.

This grilled chicken and steamed broccoli dish is an excellent choice for adults with type 1 diabetes. The lean protein from the chicken, combined with the fiber and nutrients from the broccoli, makes for a well-balanced and diabetes-friendly meal.

The simple seasoning and lemon juice add flavor without adding significant carbohydrates. You can adjust the portion sizes as needed to fit your individual carb and calorie requirements.

To make this meal even more satisfying, you can serve it with a side of roasted or sautéed low-carb vegetables, such as zucchini or cauliflower.

3. Spaghetti Squash with Meatballs

Ingredients: **Dinner**

- 1 medium spaghetti squash,
halved lengthwise and seeded
- 1 lb ground turkey or lean ground beef
- 1/2 cup grated Parmesan cheese
- 1/4 cup breadcrumbs
- 1 egg, lightly beaten
- 2 cloves garlic, minced
- 1 tsp dried oregano
- 1/2 tsp salt
- 1/4 tsp black pepper
- 1 (24 oz) jar marinara sauce

PreparationTime: 20 minutes
Cook Time: 45 minutes
Total Time: 1 hour 5 minutes
Serves: 4

↓↓↓

1. Preheat the oven to 400°F. Line a baking sheet with parchment paper.

2. Place the spaghetti squash halves cut-side down on the prepared baking sheet. Bake for 35-45 minutes, until the squash is tender when pierced with a fork.

3. In a medium bowl, combine the ground turkey or beef, Parmesan cheese, breadcrumbs, egg, garlic, oregano, salt, and black pepper. Mix well and form into 12-16 meatballs.

4. In a large skillet, cook the meatballs over medium heat, turning occasionally, until browned on all sides and cooked through, about 8-10 minutes.

5. Remove the spaghetti squash from the oven and use a fork to shred the flesh into spaghetti-like strands.

6. Divide the spaghetti squash strands among 4 plates or bowls. Top each portion with 3-4 meatballs and a generous amount of marinara sauce. Serve immediately.

This spaghetti squash with meatballs dish is a great low-carb alternative to traditional pasta. The spaghetti squash provides a similar texture and flavor, while the meatballs and marinara sauce add protein and flavor.

You can use either ground turkey or lean ground beef for the meatballs, depending on your preference. Adjust the portion sizes as needed to fit your individual dietary needs.

4. Stuffed Zucchini Boats with Ground Turkey

Ingredients:

- 4 medium zucchini, halved lengthwise
- 1 lb ground turkey
- 1/2 cup diced onion
- 2 cloves garlic, minced
- 1 tsp dried oregano
- 1/2 tsp dried basil
- 1/4 tsp red pepper flakes (optional)
- 1/2 tsp salt
- 1/4 tsp black pepper
- 1 cup shredded mozzarella cheese
- 2 tbsp grated Parmesan cheese
- Chopped fresh parsley for garnish (optional)

Dinner

PreparationTime: 20 minutes
Cook Time: 30 minutes
Total Time: 50 minutes
Serves: 4

↓↓

1. Preheat the oven to 375°F. Lightly grease a baking dish.

2. Using a spoon or melon baller, scoop out the flesh from the center of each zucchini half, leaving a 1/4-inch shell. Chop the scooped-out zucchini flesh.

3. In a skillet over medium heat, cook the ground turkey, diced onion, and minced garlic until the turkey is browned and the onion is translucent, about 5-7 minutes. Drain any excess fat.

4. Stir in the chopped zucchini flesh, dried oregano, dried basil, red pepper flakes (if using), salt, and black pepper. Cook for an additional 2-3 minutes.

5. Arrange the zucchini boats in the prepared baking dish. Spoon the turkey mixture evenly into the zucchini boats.

6. Top each stuffed zucchini boat with shredded mozzarella cheese and grated Parmesan cheese.

7. Bake for 25-30 minutes, until the zucchini is tender and the cheese is melted and bubbly.

8. Garnish with chopped fresh parsley, if desired.

9. Serve hot.

This stuffed zucchini boat recipe is a great low-carb and protein-packed meal option. The ground turkey filling provides a satisfying and flavorful topping for the roasted zucchini boats.

You can adjust the spices and cheese toppings to your personal preferences. Serve this dish with a side salad or roasted vegetables for a complete and balanced meal.

5. Cauliflower Rice Stir-Fry

Ingredients:

Dinner

- 1 head of cauliflower, riced or finely chopped
- 1 tbsp olive oil
- 1 lb boneless, skinless chicken breasts, cut into 1-inch pieces
- 1 red bell pepper, sliced
- 1 cup broccoli florets
- 1 cup sliced mushrooms
- 2 cloves garlic, minced
- 1 tbsp grated fresh ginger
- 2 tbsp low-sodium soy sauce
- 1 tbsp rice vinegar
- 1 tsp sesame oil
- 1/4 tsp red pepper flakes (optional)
- Salt and black pepper to taste
- Chopped green onions for garnish (optional)

PreparationTime: 15 minutes
Cook Time: 15 minutes
Total Time: 30 minutes
Serves: 4

↓↓

1. In a food processor, pulse the cauliflower florets until they resemble rice-sized grains. Set aside.

2. Heat the olive oil in a large skillet or wok over medium-high heat. Add the chicken and cook for 5-7 minutes, stirring occasionally, until the chicken is lightly browned.

3. Add the sliced bell pepper, broccoli florets, and mushrooms to the skillet. Cook for an additional 3-5 minutes, until the vegetables are tender-crisp.

4. Stir in the minced garlic and grated ginger. Cook for 1 minute, until fragrant.

5. Add the riced cauliflower, soy sauce, rice vinegar, and sesame oil to the skillet. Toss everything together and cook for 3-5 minutes, until the cauliflower rice is tender.

6. If using, sprinkle the red pepper flakes over the stir-fry.

7. Season with salt and black pepper to taste.

8. Serve the cauliflower rice stir-fry hot, garnished with chopped green onions if desired.

This cauliflower rice stir-fry is a great option for adults with type 1 diabetes as it is low in carbs, high in protein, and packed with fiber and nutrients from the vegetables. The combination of chicken, cauliflower rice, and stir-fried veggies makes for a satisfying and balanced meal.

Adjust the portion sizes as needed to fit your individual carb and calorie requirements. You can also customize the vegetables used based on your preferences.

6. Beef and Vegetable Stew

Dinner

Ingredients:

PreparationTime: 20 minutes
Cook Time: 1 hour 30 minutes
Total Time: 1 hour 50 minutes
Serves: 6

- 1 lb beef stew meat, cut into 1-inch cubes
- 2 tbsp olive oil
- 1 medium onion, diced
- 3 cloves garlic, minced
- 2 cups low-sodium beef broth
- 1 (14.5 oz) can diced tomatoes
- 2 medium carrots, peeled and sliced
- 2 medium potatoes, peeled and cubed
- 1 cup frozen green beans
- 1 tsp dried thyme
- 1 tsp dried rosemary
- 1/2 tsp salt
- 1/4 tsp black pepper

↓↓

1. In a large pot or Dutch oven, heat the olive oil over medium-high heat. Add the beef cubes and brown on all sides, about 5-7 minutes. Remove the beef from the pot and set aside.

2. Add the diced onion to the pot and cook for 3-4 minutes, until translucent. Add the minced garlic and cook for an additional minute, stirring constantly.

3. Pour in the beef broth and diced tomatoes, scraping up any browned bits from the bottom of the pot.

4. Add the browned beef, sliced carrots, cubed potatoes, frozen green beans, dried thyme, dried rosemary, salt, and black pepper. Stir to combine.

5. Bring the stew to a boil, then reduce the heat to low, cover, and simmer for 1 to 1.5 hours, or until the beef and vegetables are tender.

6. Taste and adjust seasoning as needed.

7. Serve the beef and vegetable stew hot.

This beef and vegetable stew is a great option for adults with type 1 diabetes as it is high in protein, fiber, and complex carbohydrates, while being relatively low in simple carbs. The combination of lean beef, vegetables, and a flavorful broth makes for a satisfying and nutrient-dense meal. Be sure to adjust portion sizes as needed to fit your individual carb and calorie requirements. You can also customize the vegetables used based on your preferences.

7. Baked Tilapia with Roasted Vegetables

Ingredients:

- 4 (6 oz) tilapia fillets
- 2 tbsp olive oil, divided
- 1 tsp lemon zest
- 1 tbsp lemon juice
- 1 tsp dried dill
- 1/4 tsp salt
- 1/4 tsp black pepper
- 1 medium zucchini, sliced
- 1 medium yellow squash, sliced
- 1 red bell pepper, sliced
- 1 cup broccoli florets
- 2 cloves garlic, minced
- 1 tbsp chopped fresh parsley (optional)

Dinner

PreparationTime: 20 minutes
Cook Time: 30 minutes
Total Time: 50 minutes
Serves: 4

↓↓

1. Preheat the oven to 400°F. Line a large baking sheet with parchment paper.

2. In a small bowl, combine 1 tbsp of the olive oil, lemon zest, lemon juice, dried dill, salt, and black pepper. Brush this mixture over the top of the tilapia fillets.

3. Arrange the tilapia fillets on one side of the prepared baking sheet.

4. In a large bowl, toss the sliced zucchini, yellow squash, bell pepper, and broccoli florets with the remaining 1 tbsp of olive oil and the minced garlic. Season with a pinch of salt and pepper.

5. Spread the seasoned vegetables in a single layer on the other side of the baking sheet, next to the tilapia.

6. Bake for 25-30 minutes, or until the fish flakes easily with a fork and the vegetables are tender.

7. Garnish the baked tilapia and roasted vegetables with chopped fresh parsley, if desired.

8. Serve immediately.

This baked tilapia and roasted vegetable dish is an excellent choice for adults with type 1 diabetes. The lean protein from the tilapia, combined with the fiber and nutrients from the roasted vegetables, makes for a well-balanced and diabetes-friendly meal.

The lemon and dill seasoning on the tilapia adds flavor without adding significant carbohydrates. Adjust the portion sizes as needed to fit your individual carb and calorie requirements.

8. Chicken and Spinach Stuffed Portobello Mushrooms

Ingredients:

- 4 large portobello mushroom caps,
stems removed and chopped
- 1 tbsp olive oil
- 1 lb boneless, skinless chicken breasts, diced
- 2 cloves garlic, minced
- 1 cup baby spinach, chopped
- 1/4 cup grated Parmesan cheese
- 2 tbsp cream cheese, softened
- 1/4 tsp salt
- 1/4 tsp black pepper

Dinner

PreparationTime: 20 minutes
Cook Time: 25 minutes
Total Time: 45 minutes
Serves: 4

↓↓↓

1. Preheat the oven to 400°F. Lightly grease a baking sheet or line it with parchment paper.

2. Arrange the portobello mushroom caps, gill-side up, on the prepared baking sheet.

3. In a skillet over medium heat, heat the olive oil. Add the chopped mushroom stems, diced chicken, and minced garlic. Cook for 5-7 minutes, until the chicken is cooked through.

4. Remove the skillet from heat and stir in the chopped spinach, Parmesan cheese, cream cheese, salt, and black pepper. Mix well until the cheese is melted and the ingredients are combined.

5. Spoon the chicken and spinach mixture evenly into the portobello mushroom caps.

6. Bake for 20-25 minutes, until the mushrooms are tender and the filling is hot and bubbly.

7. Serve the stuffed portobello mushrooms immediately.

This chicken and spinach stuffed portobello mushroom dish is a great option for adults with type 1 diabetes. The portobello mushroom caps provide a low-carb "vessel" for the protein-rich chicken and nutrient-dense spinach filling.

The combination of lean protein, healthy fats, and fiber makes this a well-balanced and satisfying meal. Adjust the portion sizes as needed to fit your individual carb and calorie requirements.

You can also try substituting the chicken with ground turkey or tofu for a vegetarian option.

9. Turkey Meatloaf with a Side Salad

Ingredients:

Dinner

Turkey Meatloaf:
- 1 lb ground turkey
- 1/2 cup whole wheat breadcrumbs
- 1/4 cup diced onion
- 1 egg, lightly beaten
- 2 tbsp tomato paste
- 1 tsp dried oregano
- 1/2 tsp garlic powder
- 1/4 tsp salt
- 1/4 tsp black pepper

Side Salad:
- 6 cups mixed greens
- 1 cup cherry tomatoes, halved
- 1/2 cucumber, sliced
- 2 tbsp olive oil
- 1 tbsp balsamic vinegar
- 1 tsp Dijon mustard
- 1/4 tsp salt
- 1/4 tsp black pepper

PreparationTime: 20 minutes
Cook Time: 1 hour
Total Time: 1 hour 20 minutes
Serves: 6

↓↓

Turkey Meatloaf:
1. Preheat the oven to 375°F. Lightly grease a 9x5-inch loaf pan.
2. In a large bowl, combine the ground turkey, breadcrumbs, diced onion, egg, tomato paste, oregano, garlic powder, salt, and black pepper. Mix well until fully incorporated.
3. Transfer the turkey mixture to the prepared loaf pan and shape it into a loaf.
4. Bake for 55-60 minutes, or until the internal temperature reaches 165°F.
5. Let the meatloaf rest for 5 minutes before slicing and serving.

Side Salad:
1. In a large salad bowl, combine the mixed greens, cherry tomatoes, and sliced cucumber.
2. In a small bowl, whisk together the olive oil, balsamic vinegar, Dijon mustard, salt, and black pepper to make the dressing.
3. Drizzle the dressing over the salad and toss gently to coat.

Serve the sliced turkey meatloaf with the side salad. This meal is a great option for adults with type 1 diabetes as it is high in protein, low in carbs, and provides a good source of fiber and nutrients from the salad.

Adjust the portion sizes as needed to fit your individual carb and calorie requirements. You can also customize the salad ingredients based on your preferences.

10. Lentil and Vegetable Curry

Ingredients:

Dinner

PreparationTime: 20 minutes
Cook Time: 30 minutes
Total Time: 50 minutes
Serves: 4

- 1 cup dry brown or green lentils, rinsed
- 2 cups low-sodium vegetable broth
- 1 tbsp olive oil
- 1 medium onion, diced
- 3 cloves garlic, minced
- 1 tbsp grated fresh ginger
- 1 tsp garam masala
- 1 tsp ground cumin
- 1 tsp ground coriander
- 1/2 tsp turmeric
- 1/4 tsp cayenne pepper (optional)
- 1 (14 oz) can diced tomatoes
- 1 cup cauliflower florets
- 1 cup diced zucchini
- 1 cup diced bell pepper
- 1/4 cup chopped fresh cilantro
- 1/4 tsp salt
- 1/4 tsp black pepper

↓↓↓

1. In a medium saucepan, combine the rinsed lentils and vegetable broth. Bring to a boil, then reduce heat and simmer for 15-20 minutes, until the lentils are tender. Drain any excess liquid and set aside.

2. In a large skillet or Dutch oven, heat the olive oil over medium heat. Add the diced onion and cook for 3-4 minutes, until translucent.

3. Stir in the minced garlic, grated ginger, garam masala, cumin, coriander, turmeric, and cayenne pepper (if using). Cook for 1 minute, until fragrant.

4. Add the diced tomatoes, cauliflower florets, diced zucchini, and diced bell pepper. Stir to combine.

5. Stir in the cooked lentils and chopped fresh cilantro. Season with salt and black pepper.

6. Reduce heat to low and simmer the curry for 10-15 minutes, until the vegetables are tender. Serve the lentil and vegetable curry hot, over cauliflower rice or with a side of steamed greens.

This lentil and vegetable curry is a great option for adults with type 1 diabetes. The lentils provide a good source of protein and fiber, while the vegetables add vitamins, minerals, and antioxidants. The spices add flavor without significantly increasing the carb content. Adjust the portion sizes as needed to fit your individual carb and calorie requirements. You can also customize the vegetables used based on your preferences.

11. Chicken Fajitas with Bell Peppers

Ingredients:

- 1 lb boneless,
skinless chicken breasts, sliced into thin strips
- 2 bell peppers (any color), sliced into thin strips
- 1 onion, sliced into thin strips
- 2 tbsp olive oil
- 2 tsp chili powder
- 1 tsp cumin
- 1 tsp garlic powder
- 1 tsp oregano
- Salt and pepper to taste
- 8 flour tortillas
- Toppings (optional): shredded cheese, sour cream, guacamole, salsa

Dinner

PreparationTime: 20 minutes
Cook Time: 20 minutes
Total Time: 40 minutes
Serves: 4

↓↓↓

1. In a large skillet or wok, heat the olive oil over medium-high heat.

2. Add the chicken, bell peppers, and onion to the skillet. Season with the chili powder, cumin, garlic powder, oregano, salt, and pepper.

3. Cook, stirring occasionally, for 15-20 minutes or until the chicken is cooked through and the vegetables are tender.

4. Warm the flour tortillas according to package instructions.

5. Serve the chicken fajita mixture in the warm tortillas. Top with desired toppings such as shredded cheese, sour cream, guacamole, and salsa.

Enjoy your Chicken Fajitas with Bell Peppers! This dish is perfect for a quick and easy weeknight meal.

12. Eggplant Parmesan with a Side Salad

Ingredients:

- 2 medium eggplants, sliced into 1/2-inch thick rounds
- 2 eggs, beaten
- 1 cup breadcrumbs
- 1 cup grated Parmesan cheese
- 1 jar (24 oz) marinara sauce
- 8 oz shredded mozzarella cheese

Side Salad Ingredients:
- 5 oz mixed greens
- 1 tomato, diced
- 1/2 cucumber, sliced
- 2 tbsp olive oil
- 1 tbsp balsamic vinegar
- Salt and pepper to taste

Dinner

PreparationTime: 20 minutes
Cook Time: 45 minutes
Total Time: 1 hour 5 minutes
Serves: 4

Eggplant Parmesan

↓↓↓

Eggplant Parmesan:
1. Preheat oven to 375°F. Grease a baking sheet.
2. Dip the eggplant slices in the beaten eggs, then coat in the breadcrumb-Parmesan mixture.
3. Arrange the breaded eggplant slices in a single layer on the prepared baking sheet.
4. Bake for 20-25 minutes, flipping halfway, until golden brown.
5. Spread a layer of marinara sauce in the bottom of a 9x13 inch baking dish. Arrange the baked eggplant slices in a single layer. Top with the remaining marinara sauce and the shredded mozzarella cheese.
6. Bake for 20-25 minutes until the cheese is melted and bubbly.

Side Salad:
1. In a large bowl, combine the mixed greens, tomato, and cucumber.
2. Drizzle the olive oil and balsamic vinegar over the salad and toss to coat.
3. Season with salt and pepper to taste.

Serve the Eggplant Parmesan hot, with the side salad on the side. Enjoy!

13. Grilled Pork Chops with Brussels Sprouts

Ingredients:

- 4 boneless pork chops (about 4-6 oz each)
- 1 lb Brussels sprouts, trimmed and halved
- 2 tbsp olive oil
- 1 tsp garlic powder
- 1 tsp dried thyme
- Salt and pepper to taste
- Lemon wedges for serving

Dinner

PreparationTime: 15 minutes
Cook Time: 25 minutes
Total Time: 40 minutes
Serves: 4

↓↓

1. Preheat grill or grill pan to medium-high heat.

2. In a large bowl, toss the Brussels sprouts with 1 tbsp of the olive oil, garlic powder, thyme, salt, and pepper.

3. Spread the Brussels sprouts on a baking sheet and roast in the preheated oven for 18-22 minutes, stirring halfway, until tender and lightly browned.

4. Brush the pork chops with the remaining 1 tbsp of olive oil and season with salt and pepper.

5. Grill the pork chops for 4-5 minutes per side, or until they reach an internal temperature of 145°F.

6. Let the pork chops rest for 5 minutes before serving.

7. Serve the grilled pork chops with the roasted Brussels sprouts and lemon wedges.

Nutritional Information (per serving):
- Calories: 300 - Total Carbs: 12g
- Fiber: 4g - Net Carbs: 8g - Protein: 32g - Fat: 15g

This recipe is suitable for adults with type 1 diabetes as it is low in carbs and provides a balanced meal with lean protein, fiber-rich vegetables, and healthy fats. The portion sizes and nutrient profile can help manage blood sugar levels. As always, consult with your healthcare team for personalized dietary recommendations.

14. Mushroom and Spinach Stuffed Chicken Breast

Ingredients:

Dinner

- 4 boneless, skinless chicken breasts (about 6 oz each)
- 8 oz mushrooms, sliced
- 2 cups fresh spinach, chopped
- 2 cloves garlic, minced
- 2 tbsp cream cheese, softened
- 1/4 cup grated Parmesan cheese
- 1 tsp dried thyme
- Salt and pepper to taste
- 1 tbsp olive oil

PreparationTime: 20 minutes
Cook Time: 30 minutes
Total Time: 50 minutes
Serves: 4

↓↓

1. Preheat oven to 375°F.

2. In a skillet over medium heat, sauté the mushrooms and garlic in the olive oil for 5-7 minutes, until mushrooms are tender. Add the spinach and cook for 2-3 minutes until wilted. Remove from heat and let cool slightly.

3. In a small bowl, mix the sautéed mushroom-spinach mixture with the cream cheese and Parmesan cheese. Season with thyme, salt, and pepper.

4. Slice the chicken breasts horizontally to create a pocket. Stuff each chicken breast with the mushroom-spinach mixture, dividing it evenly.

5. Place the stuffed chicken breasts in a baking dish and bake for 25-30 minutes, or until the chicken is cooked through and reaches an internal temperature of 165°F. Serve the stuffed chicken breasts immediately.

Nutritional Information (per serving):
- Calories: 280
- Total Carbs: 5g
- Fiber: 1g
- Net Carbs: 4g
- Protein: 40g
- Fat: 12g

This recipe is suitable for adults with type 1 diabetes as it is low in carbs and provides a balanced meal with lean protein, fiber-rich vegetables, and healthy fats. The portion sizes and nutrient profile can help manage blood sugar levels. As always, consult with your healthcare team for personalized dietary recommendations.

15. Quinoa and Vegetable Stir-Fry

Ingredients: **Dinner**

PreparationTime: 15 minutes
Cook Time: 20 minutes
Total Time: 35 minutes
Serves: 4

- 1 cup uncooked quinoa, rinsed
- 2 cups low-sodium vegetable broth
- 1 tbsp sesame oil
- 2 cloves garlic, minced
- 1 inch piece fresh ginger, grated
- 1 red bell pepper, sliced
- 1 cup broccoli florets
- 1 cup sliced mushrooms
- 1 cup snow peas or snap peas
- 2 cups baby spinach
- 2 tbsp low-sodium soy sauce or tamari
- 1 tsp sesame seeds (optional)
- Salt and pepper to taste

↓↓

1. In a medium saucepan, combine the quinoa and vegetable broth. Bring to a boil, then reduce heat to low, cover, and simmer for 15-20 minutes, until quinoa is cooked and liquid is absorbed.

2. In a large skillet or wok, heat the sesame oil over medium-high heat. Add the garlic and ginger and cook for 1 minute, until fragrant.

3. Add the bell pepper, broccoli, mushrooms, and snow peas to the skillet. Stir-fry for 5-7 minutes, until vegetables are tender-crisp.

4. Stir in the cooked quinoa, baby spinach, and soy sauce. Cook for 2-3 minutes, until the spinach is wilted.

5. Remove from heat and season with salt and pepper to taste. Serve the quinoa and vegetable stir-fry warm, garnished with sesame seeds if desired.

Nutritional Information (per serving):
- Calories: 250
- Total Carbs: 35g
- Fiber: 6g
- Net Carbs: 29g
- Protein: 10g
- Fat: 8g

This recipe is suitable for adults with type 1 diabetes as it is moderate in carbs and provides a balanced meal with complex carbohydrates, fiber-rich vegetables, and healthy fats. The portion sizes and nutrient profile can help manage blood sugar levels. As always, consult with your healthcare team for personalized dietary recommendations.

16. Baked Cod with Lemon and Herbs

Ingredients:

- 4 (6 oz) cod fillets
- 2 tbsp olive oil
- 2 tbsp freshly squeezed lemon juice
- 2 tsp grated lemon zest
- 2 cloves garlic, minced
- 2 tbsp chopped fresh parsley
- 1 tbsp chopped fresh dill
- 1/4 tsp salt
- 1/4 tsp black pepper

Dinner

PreparationTime: 10 minutes
Cook Time: 20 minutes
Total Time: 30 minutes
Serves: 4

↓↓↓

1. Preheat oven to 400°F. Grease a baking dish or line it with parchment paper.

2. In a small bowl, whisk together the olive oil, lemon juice, lemon zest, garlic, parsley, dill, salt, and pepper.

3. Place the cod fillets in the prepared baking dish. Pour the lemon-herb mixture over the top, making sure to evenly coat the fish.

4. Bake for 18-22 minutes, or until the cod is opaque and flakes easily with a fork.

5. Serve the baked cod immediately, garnished with additional lemon wedges and fresh herbs if desired.

Nutritional Information (per serving):
- Calories: 200
- Total Carbs: 2g
- Fiber: 0g
- Net Carbs: 2g
- Protein: 30g
- Fat: 8g

This recipe is suitable for adults with type 1 diabetes as it is very low in carbs and provides a balanced meal with lean protein, healthy fats, and minimal carbohydrates. The portion sizes and nutrient profile can help manage blood sugar levels. As always, consult with your healthcare team for personalized dietary recommendations.

17. Chili Lime Chicken with Cauliflower Rice

Ingredients:

Dinner

- 1 lb boneless, skinless chicken breasts, cut into 1-inch cubes
- 2 tbsp olive oil
- 2 tsp chili powder
- 1 tsp ground cumin
- 1 tsp garlic powder
- 1 tsp dried oregano
- 1 tsp grated lime zest
- 2 tbsp freshly squeezed lime juice
- Salt and pepper to taste
- 4 cups riced cauliflower (about 1 medium head)
- 2 tbsp chopped fresh cilantro (optional)

Preparation Time: 15 minutes
Cook Time: 25 minutes
Total Time: 40 minutes
Serves: 4

↓↓

1. In a large bowl, combine the chicken, olive oil, chili powder, cumin, garlic powder, oregano, lime zest, lime juice, salt, and pepper. Toss to coat the chicken evenly.

2. Heat a large skillet or wok over medium-high heat. Add the seasoned chicken and cook for 8-10 minutes, stirring occasionally, until the chicken is cooked through and no longer pink.

3. Add the riced cauliflower to the skillet and continue cooking for 5-7 minutes, stirring frequently, until the cauliflower is tender and heated through.

4. Remove from heat and stir in the chopped cilantro, if using. Serve the chili lime chicken and cauliflower rice immediately.

Nutritional Information (per serving):
- Calories: 250
- Total Carbs: 10g
- Fiber: 4g
- Net Carbs: 6g
- Protein: 30g
- Fat: 10g

This recipe is suitable for adults with type 1 diabetes as it is low in carbs and provides a balanced meal with lean protein, fiber-rich vegetables, and healthy fats. The portion sizes and nutrient profile can help manage blood sugar levels. As always, consult with your healthcare team for personalized dietary recommendations.

18. Stuffed Bell Peppers with Quinoa and Beans

Ingredients:

Dinner

PreparationTime: 20 minutes
Cook Time: 40 minutes
Total Time: 1 hour
Serves: 4

- 4 medium bell peppers, halved and seeded
- 1 cup cooked quinoa
- 1 (15 oz) can black beans, rinsed and drained
- 1 cup diced tomatoes
- 1/2 cup shredded cheddar cheese
- 2 tbsp chopped fresh cilantro
- 1 tsp chili powder
- 1/2 tsp cumin
- 1/4 tsp garlic powder
- Salt and pepper to taste

↓↓↓

1. Preheat oven to 375°F. Grease a baking dish or line it with parchment paper.

2. In a large bowl, combine the cooked quinoa, black beans, diced tomatoes, 1/4 cup of the shredded cheese, cilantro, chili powder, cumin, garlic powder, salt, and pepper. Mix well.

3. Stuff the bell pepper halves evenly with the quinoa and bean mixture.

4. Place the stuffed bell peppers in the prepared baking dish. Top with the remaining 1/4 cup of shredded cheese.

5. Bake for 35-40 minutes, or until the peppers are tender and the cheese is melted and bubbly.

6. Serve the stuffed bell peppers warm.

Nutritional Information (per serving):
- Calories: 250 - Total Carbs: 35g - Fiber: 9g - Net Carbs: 26g
- Protein: 14g - Fat: 8g

This recipe is suitable for adults with type 1 diabetes as it is moderate in carbs and provides a balanced meal with complex carbohydrates, fiber-rich vegetables, and plant-based protein. The portion sizes and nutrient profile can help manage blood sugar levels. As always, consult with your healthcare team for personalized dietary recommendations.

19. Broccoli and Cheddar Stuffed Chicken

Ingredients:

Dinner

- 4 boneless, skinless chicken breasts (about 6 oz each)
- 1 cup chopped broccoli florets
- 1/2 cup shredded cheddar cheese
- 2 tbsp cream cheese, softened
- 1 tsp garlic powder
- 1/2 tsp dried thyme
- Salt and pepper to taste
- 1 tbsp olive oil

PreparationTime: 20 minutes
Cook Time: 30 minutes
Total Time: 50 minutes
Serves: 4

↓↓

1. Preheat oven to 375°F. Grease a baking dish or line it with parchment paper.

2. Slice each chicken breast horizontally to create a pocket, being careful not to cut all the way through.

3. In a medium bowl, mix together the chopped broccoli, cheddar cheese, cream cheese, garlic powder, and thyme. Season with salt and pepper.

4. Stuff the broccoli and cheese mixture evenly into the pockets of the chicken breasts.

5. Heat the olive oil in a large oven-safe skillet over medium-high heat. Add the stuffed chicken breasts and sear for 2-3 minutes per side to create a golden-brown crust.

6. Transfer the skillet to the preheated oven and bake for 20-25 minutes, or until the chicken is cooked through and reaches an internal temperature of 165°F.

7. Serve the broccoli and cheddar stuffed chicken immediately.

Nutritional Information (per serving):
- Calories: 280 - Total Carbs: 6g - Fiber: 2g - Net Carbs: 4g - Protein: 35g
- Fat: 13g

This recipe is suitable for adults with type 1 diabetes as it is low in carbs and provides a balanced meal with lean protein, fiber-rich vegetables, and healthy fats. The portion sizes and nutrient profile can help manage blood sugar levels. As always, consult with your healthcare team for personalized dietary recommendations.

20. Vegetable and Chickpea Tagine

Ingredients:

Dinner

- 1 tbsp olive oil
- 1 onion, diced
- 3 cloves garlic, minced
- 1 tsp ground cumin
- 1 tsp ground coriander
- 1 tsp paprika
- 1/2 tsp ground cinnamon
- 1/4 tsp cayenne pepper (or to taste)
- 1 (15 oz) can chickpeas, rinsed and drained
- 1 (14 oz) can diced tomatoes
- 1 cup low-sodium vegetable broth
- 2 cups diced butternut squash
- 1 cup cauliflower florets
- 1 cup green beans, trimmed and cut into 1-inch pieces
- 1/4 cup chopped fresh cilantro
- Salt and pepper to taste

PreparationTime: 20 minutes
Cook Time: 40 minutes
Total Time: 1 hour
Serves: 4

↓↓

1. In a large pot or Dutch oven, heat the olive oil over medium heat. Add the onion and sauté for 5 minutes until translucent.

2. Add the garlic, cumin, coriander, paprika, cinnamon, and cayenne. Cook for 1 minute, stirring constantly, until fragrant.

3. Stir in the chickpeas, diced tomatoes, and vegetable broth. Bring the mixture to a simmer.

4. Add the butternut squash, cauliflower, and green beans. Reduce heat to medium-low, cover, and simmer for 30-35 minutes, or until the vegetables are tender.

5. Remove from heat and stir in the chopped cilantro. Season with salt and pepper to taste.

6. Serve the vegetable and chickpea tagine warm.

Nutritional Information (per serving):
- Calories: 250 - Total Carbs: 35g - Fiber: 9g - Net Carbs: 26g
- Protein: 10g - Fat: 7g

This recipe is suitable for adults with type 1 diabetes as it is moderate in carbs and provides a balanced meal with complex carbohydrates, fiber-rich vegetables, and plant-based protein. The portion sizes and nutrient profile can help manage blood sugar levels. As always, consult with your healthcare team for personalized dietary recommendations.

1. Celery Sticks with Almond Butter

Ingredients:

- 3-4 celery stalks, cut into 3-inch sticks
- 2 tbsp unsweetened almond butter

PreparationTime: 5 minutes
Total Time: 5 minutes
Serves: 1

↓↓↓

1. Wash and cut the celery stalks into 3-inch sticks.

2. Spread 1-2 teaspoons of almond butter onto each celery stick.

Nutritional Information (per serving):
- Calories: 150
- Total Carbs: 6g
- Fiber: 3g
- Net Carbs: 3g
- Protein: 5g
- Fat: 12g

This snack is an excellent choice for adults with type 1 diabetes as it is low in carbs and provides a good source of healthy fats and fiber. The combination of celery and almond butter can help manage blood sugar levels and provide a satisfying snack.

Some key benefits of this recipe for type 1 diabetes:

- Low in carbs: The net carb count is only 3g per serving, which is ideal for managing blood sugar.
- High in fiber: The celery provides 3g of fiber, which can help slow the absorption of carbs.
- Good source of healthy fats: The almond butter provides heart-healthy monounsaturated fats.
- Portable and easy to prepare: This snack can be easily packed for on-the-go.

As always, be sure to consult with your healthcare team for personalized dietary recommendations.

2. Greek Yogurt with a Sprinkle of Nuts

Ingredients:

- 1 cup plain, unsweetened Greek yogurt
- 2 tbsp chopped nuts
(such as almonds, walnuts, or pecans)

Snacks

PreparationTime: 5 minutes
Total Time: 5 minutes
Serves: 1

↓↓

1. Scoop the Greek yogurt into a bowl.

2. Sprinkle the chopped nuts over the top of the yogurt.

Nutritional Information (per serving):
- Calories: 200
- Total Carbs: 10g
- Fiber: 2g
- Net Carbs: 8g
- Protein: 20g
- Fat: 10g

This snack is an excellent choice for adults with type 1 diabetes as it is moderate in carbs and provides a good balance of protein, healthy fats, and fiber. The combination of Greek yogurt and nuts can help manage blood sugar levels and provide a satisfying snack.

Some key benefits of this recipe for type 1 diabetes:

- Moderate in carbs: The net carb count is 8g per serving, which is a reasonable amount for a snack.
- High in protein: The Greek yogurt provides 20g of protein, which can help stabilize blood sugar.
- Good source of healthy fats: The nuts provide heart-healthy monounsaturated and polyunsaturated fats.
- Fiber-rich: The nuts add 2g of fiber, which can help slow the absorption of carbs.

As always, be sure to consult with your healthcare team for personalized dietary recommendations.

3. Hummus with Sliced Cucumbers

Ingredients:

- 2 tbsp homemade or
 store-bought unsweetened hummus
- 1 cup sliced cucumber

PreparationTime: 5 minutes
Total Time: 5 minutes
Serves: 1

↓↓

1. Scoop the hummus into a small bowl or ramekin.

2. Arrange the sliced cucumber around the hummus.

Nutritional Information (per serving):
- Calories: 100
- Total Carbs: 10g
- Fiber: 3g
- Net Carbs: 7g
- Protein: 4g
- Fat: 6g

This snack is an excellent choice for adults with type 1 diabetes as it is low in carbs and provides a good balance of protein, healthy fats, and fiber. The combination of hummus and cucumbers can help manage blood sugar levels and provide a satisfying snack.

Some key benefits of this recipe for type 1 diabetes:

- Low in carbs: The net carb count is only 7g per serving, which is ideal for managing blood sugar.
- High in fiber: The cucumbers provide 3g of fiber, which can help slow the absorption of carbs.
- Good source of protein and healthy fats: The hummus provides plant-based protein and unsaturated fats.
- Hydrating and refreshing: The cucumbers are high in water content, which can help with hydration.

As always, be sure to consult with your healthcare team for personalized dietary recommendations.

4. Apple Slices with Peanut Butter

Ingredients:

- 1 medium apple, cored and sliced
- 2 tbsp natural, unsweetened peanut butter

PreparationTime: 5 minutes
Total Time: 5 minutes
Serves: 1

↓↓↓

1. Wash and slice the apple into thin wedges.

2. Spread 1-2 teaspoons of peanut butter onto each apple slice.

Nutritional Information (per serving):
- Calories: 180
- Total Carbs: 16g
- Fiber: 4g
- Net Carbs: 12g
- Protein: 7g
- Fat: 10g

This snack is a good choice for adults with type 1 diabetes as it provides a balance of carbohydrates, protein, and healthy fats. The combination of apple and peanut butter can help manage blood sugar levels and provide a satisfying snack.

Some key benefits of this recipe for type 1 diabetes:

- Moderate in carbs: The net carb count is 12g per serving, which is a reasonable amount for a snack.
- Good source of fiber: The apple provides 4g of fiber, which can help slow the absorption of carbs.
- Provides protein and healthy fats: The peanut butter adds protein and unsaturated fats to help stabilize blood sugar.
- Portable and easy to prepare: This snack can be easily packed for on-the-go.

As always, be sure to consult with your healthcare team for personalized dietary recommendations.

5. Mixed Nuts and Seeds

Ingredients:

- 1/4 cup mixed nuts (such as almonds, walnuts, pecans)   **PreparationTime: 5 minutes**
- 1 tbsp mixed seeds (such as pumpkin, sunflower, chia, flax)   **Total Time: 5 minutes**

Serves: 1

↓↓↓

1. In a small bowl or resealable bag, combine the mixed nuts and seeds.

Nutritional Information (per serving):
- Calories: 200
- Total Carbs: 6g
- Fiber: 4g
- Net Carbs: 2g
- Protein: 7g
- Fat: 18g

This mixed nuts and seeds snack is an excellent choice for adults with type 1 diabetes as it is very low in carbs and provides a good source of healthy fats, protein, and fiber.

Some key benefits of this recipe for type 1 diabetes:

- Extremely low in net carbs: With only 2g of net carbs per serving, this snack won't spike blood sugar levels.
- High in fiber: The nuts and seeds provide 4g of fiber, which can help slow the absorption of carbs.
- Good source of healthy fats: The nuts and seeds are rich in unsaturated fats, which are beneficial for heart health.
- Provides protein: The nuts and seeds offer a small amount of plant-based protein to help stabilize blood sugar.
- Portable and easy to prepare: This snack can be easily packed for on-the-go.

As always, be sure to consult with your healthcare team for personalized dietary recommendations and portion sizes.

6. Cheese Sticks

Ingredients:

- 1 oz cheddar or mozzarella cheese, cut into 4-5 sticks

Snacks

PreparationTime: 5 minutes
Total Time: 5 minutes
Serves: 1

↓↓↓

1. Cut the cheese into 4-5 stick-shaped pieces.

Nutritional Information (per serving):
- Calories: 110
- Total Carbs: 0g
- Fiber: 0g
- Net Carbs: 0g
- Protein: 7g
- Fat: 9g

This cheese stick snack is an excellent choice for adults with type 1 diabetes as it is completely carb-free and provides a good source of protein and healthy fats.

Some key benefits of this recipe for type 1 diabetes:

- Zero carbs: The cheese sticks contain no carbohydrates, making them ideal for managing blood sugar levels.
- Good source of protein: The cheese provides 7g of protein per serving, which can help stabilize blood sugar.
- Contains healthy fats: The cheese is a source of saturated and monounsaturated fats, which are beneficial for overall health.
- Portable and easy to prepare: Cheese sticks are a convenient, grab-and-go snack option.

When choosing cheese for this recipe, opt for full-fat, natural cheeses like cheddar or mozzarella, as they are more nutrient-dense and satiating compared to low-fat or processed cheese options.

As always, be sure to consult with your healthcare team for personalized dietary recommendations and portion sizes.

7. Sliced Bell Peppers with Guacamole

Ingredients:

- 1/2 medium bell pepper, sliced into strips
- 2 tbsp homemade or
 store-bought unsweetened guacamole

Snacks

PreparationTime: 10 minutes
Total Time: 10 minutes
Serves: 1

↓↓↓

1. Wash and slice the bell pepper into thin strips.

2. Scoop the guacamole into a small bowl or ramekin.

3. Dip the bell pepper strips into the guacamole and enjoy.

Nutritional Information (per serving):
- Calories: 100
- Total Carbs: 8g
- Fiber: 4g
- Net Carbs: 4g
- Protein: 2g
- Fat: 7g

This snack is an excellent choice for adults with type 1 diabetes as it is low in carbs and provides a good balance of healthy fats, fiber, and antioxidants.

Some key benefits of this recipe for type 1 diabetes:

- Low in net carbs: The net carb count is only 4g per serving, which is ideal for managing blood sugar levels.
- High in fiber: The bell peppers and guacamole provide 4g of fiber, which can help slow the absorption of carbs.
- Good source of healthy fats: The guacamole is rich in monounsaturated fats from the avocado, which can help improve insulin sensitivity.
- Provides antioxidants: Bell peppers are a great source of vitamin C and other antioxidants, which are important for overall health.
- Hydrating and refreshing: The bell peppers are high in water content, which can help with hydration.

As always, be sure to consult with your healthcare team for personalized dietary recommendations and portion sizes.

8. Hard-Boiled Eggs

Ingredients:

- 4 large eggs

Snacks

PreparationTime: 15 minutes
Cook Time: 12 minutes
Total Time: 27 minutes
Serves: 2 (2 eggs per serving)

↓↓

1. Place the eggs in a single layer in a saucepan and cover with cold water by 1 inch.

2. Bring the water to a boil over high heat. Once the water reaches a rolling boil, remove the pan from the heat and cover.

3. Let the eggs sit in the hot water for 12 minutes.

4. Drain the hot water and cover the eggs with cold water to stop the cooking process.

5. Once the eggs are cool enough to handle, peel them and enjoy.

Nutritional Information (per serving, 2 eggs):
- Calories: 140
- Total Carbs: 0g
- Fiber: 0g
- Net Carbs: 0g
- Protein: 12g
- Fat: 10g

Hard-boiled eggs are an excellent snack choice for adults with type 1 diabetes. They are completely carb-free and provide a good source of high-quality protein and healthy fats to help stabilize blood sugar levels.

Some key benefits of this recipe for type 1 diabetes:

- Zero carbs: Hard-boiled eggs contain no carbohydrates, making them ideal for managing blood sugar.
- High in protein: Each serving provides 12g of protein, which can help slow the absorption of glucose.
- Contains healthy fats: The egg yolks are a source of beneficial monounsaturated and saturated fats.
- Portable and easy to prepare: Hard-boiled eggs are a convenient, grab-and-go snack option.

As always, be sure to consult with your healthcare team for personalized dietary recommendations and portion sizes.

9. Cottage Cheese with Cherry Tomatoes

Ingredients:

- 1/2 cup low-fat or full-fat cottage cheese
- 1/2 cup cherry tomatoes, halved

Snacks

PreparationTime: 5 minutes
Total Time: 5 minutes
Serves: 1

↓↓↓

1. Scoop the cottage cheese into a small bowl.

2. Top the cottage cheese with the halved cherry tomatoes.

Nutritional Information (per serving):
- Calories: 150
- Total Carbs: 8g
- Fiber: 2g
- Net Carbs: 6g
- Protein: 18g
- Fat: 4g

This snack is an excellent choice for adults with type 1 diabetes as it provides a good balance of protein, fiber, and minimal carbs.

Some key benefits of this recipe for type 1 diabetes:

- Moderate in carbs: The net carb count is 6g per serving, which is a reasonable amount for a snack.
- High in protein: The cottage cheese provides 18g of protein, which can help stabilize blood sugar levels.
- Good source of fiber: The cherry tomatoes add 2g of fiber, which can help slow the absorption of carbs.
- Contains beneficial nutrients: Cottage cheese is a source of calcium, while cherry tomatoes provide vitamin C and other antioxidants.
- Hydrating: The high water content in the tomatoes can help with hydration.

When choosing cottage cheese, opt for a low-fat or full-fat variety, as the higher fat content can help slow the absorption of carbs and provide a more satiating snack.

As always, be sure to consult with your healthcare team for personalized dietary recommendations and portion sizes.

10. Almond Flour Crackers

Ingredients:

- 2 cups almond flour
- 1 tsp baking powder
- 1/4 tsp salt
- 1 egg
- 2 tbsp olive oil or melted coconut oil

Snacks

PreparationTime: 10 minutes
Cook Time: 12-15 minutes
Total Time: 25 minutes
Serves: 8 (4 crackers per serving)

↓↓

1. Preheat oven to 350°F. Line a baking sheet with parchment paper.

2. In a medium bowl, whisk together the almond flour, baking powder, and salt.

3. Add the egg and oil to the dry ingredients and mix until a dough forms.

4. Roll the dough out between two sheets of parchment paper to about 1/8-inch thickness.

5. Use a knife or cookie cutter to cut the dough into cracker shapes.

6. Transfer the crackers to the prepared baking sheet, spacing them apart.. Bake for 12-15 minutes, or until the crackers are golden brown and crispy. Let the crackers cool completely before serving.

Nutritional Information (per serving, 4 crackers):
- Calories: 180 - Total Carbs: 4g - Fiber: 2g - Net Carbs: 2g - Protein: 6g - Fat: 16g

These almond flour crackers are an excellent snack choice for adults with type 1 diabetes. They are low in carbs and provide a good source of healthy fats and protein to help manage blood sugar levels.

Some key benefits of this recipe for type 1 diabetes:

- Very low in net carbs: With only 2g of net carbs per serving, these crackers won't spike blood sugar.
- Good source of fiber: The almond flour provides 2g of fiber per serving, which can help slow the absorption of carbs.
- Contains healthy fats: The almond flour and oil provide beneficial monounsaturated and polyunsaturated fats.
- Satisfying and filling: The combination of protein, fiber, and healthy fats can help keep you feeling full.

As always, be sure to consult with your healthcare team for personalized dietary recommendations and portion sizes.

11. Edamame

Ingredients:

- 1 cup frozen edamame pods

↓↓

PreparationTime: 5 minutes
Cook Time: 5 minutes
Total Time: 10 minutes
Serves: 1

1. Bring a small pot of water to a boil.

2. Add the frozen edamame pods and cook for 4-5 minutes, until heated through and tender.

3. Drain the edamame and serve warm, lightly salted if desired.

Nutritional Information (per serving):
- Calories: 120
- Total Carbs: 9g
- Fiber: 5g
- Net Carbs: 4g
- Protein: 11g
- Fat: 5g

Edamame is an excellent snack choice for adults with type 1 diabetes. It is low in net carbs, high in fiber and protein, and provides a good source of nutrients.

Some key benefits of this recipe for type 1 diabetes:

- Low in net carbs: With only 4g of net carbs per serving, edamame won't significantly impact blood sugar levels.
- High in fiber: The 5g of fiber per serving can help slow the absorption of carbs.
- Good source of protein: The 11g of protein per serving can help stabilize blood sugar.
- Contains beneficial nutrients: Edamame is a source of vitamins, minerals, and antioxidants.
- Easy to prepare: Boiling frozen edamame is a quick and simple snack option.

When enjoying edamame, be mindful of portion sizes, as the carb and protein content can add up quickly. As always, consult with your healthcare team for personalized dietary recommendations.

12. Vegetable Sticks with Tzatziki

Ingredients:

- 1 cup mixed vegetable sticks
(such as cucumber, bell pepper, carrot)
- 2 tbsp homemade or
store-bought unsweetened tzatziki dip

PreparationTime: 10 minutes
Total Time: 10 minutes
Serves: 1

↓↓↓

1. Wash and cut the vegetables into thin, stick-shaped pieces.

2. Scoop the tzatziki dip into a small bowl or ramekin.

3. Dip the vegetable sticks into the tzatziki and enjoy.

Nutritional Information (per serving):
- Calories: 100
- Total Carbs: 8g
- Fiber: 3g
- Net Carbs: 5g
- Protein: 4g
- Fat: 6g

This snack is an excellent choice for adults with type 1 diabetes as it is low in carbs and provides a good balance of fiber, protein, and healthy fats.

Some key benefits of this recipe for type 1 diabetes:

- Moderate in net carbs: The 5g of net carbs per serving won't significantly impact blood sugar levels.
- High in fiber: The vegetables and tzatziki provide 3g of fiber, which can help slow the absorption of carbs.
- Good source of protein: The tzatziki dip contains protein from the Greek yogurt.
- Contains healthy fats: The tzatziki dip is made with olive oil, providing beneficial monounsaturated fats.
- Hydrating and refreshing: The vegetables are high in water content, which can help with hydration.

When choosing tzatziki, opt for a homemade or store-bought version that is unsweetened and low in added sugars. As always, consult with your healthcare team for personalized dietary recommendations and portion sizes.

13. Low-Carb Protein Bars

Ingredients: **Snacks**

- 1 cup almond flour   **PreparationTime: 15 minutes**
- 1/4 cup unsweetened whey protein powder   **Chill Time: 30 minutes**
- 1/4 cup unsweetened shredded coconut   **Total Time: 45 minutes**
- 2 tbsp unsweetened nut butter (such as almond or peanut butter)**Serves: 8 (1 bar per serving)**
- 2 tbsp unsweetened cocoa powder
- 2 tbsp granulated erythritol or other low-calorie sweetener
- 1/4 tsp salt
- 2 tbsp unsweetened almond milk

↓↓

1. Line an 8x4 inch loaf pan with parchment paper, leaving some overhang on the sides.

2. In a large bowl, mix together the almond flour, protein powder, shredded coconut, nut butter, cocoa powder, erythritol, and salt until well combined.

3. Add the almond milk and stir until a thick, fudgy dough forms.

4. Press the dough evenly into the prepared loaf pan.

5. Refrigerate for at least 30 minutes to allow the bars to firm up.

6. Lift the bars out of the pan using the parchment paper overhang. Cut into 8 equal bars.

7. Store the protein bars in the refrigerator for up to 1 week.

Nutritional Information (per serving, 1 bar):
- Calories: 130 - Total Carbs: 6g - Fiber: 3g - Net Carbs: 3g - Protein: 8g - Fat: 10g

These low-carb protein bars are an excellent snack choice for adults with type 1 diabetes. They are low in net carbs and provide a good source of protein and healthy fats to help manage blood sugar levels.

Some key benefits of this recipe for type 1 diabetes:

- Very low in net carbs: With only 3g of net carbs per bar, they won't significantly impact blood sugar.
- Good source of protein: The 8g of protein per bar can help stabilize blood sugar.
- Contains healthy fats: The almond flour and nut butter provide beneficial monounsaturated and polyunsaturated fats.
- Satisfying and filling: The combination of protein, fiber, and healthy fats can help keep you feeling full.

14. Chia Seed Pudding Cups

Ingredients:

Snacks

PreparationTime: 10 minutes
Chill Time: 2 hours
Total Time: 2 hours 10 minutes
Serves: 4 (1 cup per serving)

- 1/4 cup chia seeds
- 1 cup unsweetened almond milk
- 1 tsp vanilla extract
- 1/4 tsp ground cinnamon
- 1 tbsp unsweetened shredded coconut (optional)
- 1 tbsp chopped nuts (such as almonds or walnuts) (optional)

↓↓↓

1. In a medium bowl, whisk together the chia seeds, almond milk, vanilla extract, and cinnamon until well combined.

2. Cover the bowl and refrigerate for at least 2 hours, or up to 5 days, stirring occasionally, until the mixture has thickened to a pudding-like consistency.

3. Divide the chia seed pudding into 4 individual serving cups or containers.

4. Top each serving with a sprinkle of shredded coconut and chopped nuts, if desired.

5. Serve chilled.

Nutritional Information (per serving):
- Calories: 130 - Total Carbs: 10g - Fiber: 7g - Net Carbs: 3g - Protein: 5g - Fat: 8g

This chia seed pudding is an excellent snack choice for adults with type 1 diabetes. It is low in net carbs and provides a good source of fiber, protein, and healthy fats to help manage blood sugar levels.

Some key benefits of this recipe for type 1 diabetes:

- Very low in net carbs: With only 3g of net carbs per serving, this pudding won't significantly impact blood sugar.
- High in fiber: The 7g of fiber per serving can help slow the absorption of carbs.
- Good source of protein: The 5g of protein per serving can help stabilize blood sugar.
- Contains healthy fats: The chia seeds and optional nuts provide beneficial omega-3s and monounsaturated fats.
- Customizable: You can add your own toppings, such as berries or a sprinkle of cinnamon, to suit your preferences.

15. Baked Kale Chips

Ingredients: **Snacks**

- 1 bunch kale, stems removed   **PreparationTime: 10 minutes**
and leaves torn into bite-sized pieces   **Cook Time: 12-15 minutes**
- 1 tbsp olive oil   **Total Time: 22-25 minutes**
- 1/4 tsp salt   **Serves: 2 (about 1 cup per serving)**

↓↓

1. Preheat oven to 350°F. Line a baking sheet with parchment paper.

2. In a large bowl, toss the kale leaves with the olive oil and salt until the leaves are evenly coated.

3. Spread the kale leaves in a single layer on the prepared baking sheet.

4. Bake for 12-15 minutes, flipping the leaves halfway, until crispy and lightly browned.

5. Remove the kale chips from the oven and let cool completely before serving.

Nutritional Information (per serving, about 1 cup):
- Calories: 80 - Total Carbs: 7g
- Fiber: 2g - Net Carbs: 5g - Protein: 3g
- Fat: 5g

Baked kale chips are an excellent snack choice for adults with type 1 diabetes. They are low in net carbs and provide a good source of fiber, vitamins, and minerals.

Some key benefits of this recipe for type 1 diabetes:

- Low in net carbs: With only 5g of net carbs per serving, kale chips won't significantly impact blood sugar levels.
- High in fiber: The 2g of fiber per serving can help slow the absorption of carbs.
- Nutrient-dense: Kale is a rich source of vitamins A, C, and K, as well as antioxidants.
- Satisfying crunch: The baked kale chips provide a satisfying, crunchy texture.
- Versatile: You can experiment with different seasonings to customize the flavor.

When preparing the kale chips, be sure to remove the tough stems and thoroughly dry the leaves before baking to ensure they get crispy. As always, consult with your healthcare team for personalized dietary recommendations and portion sizes.

16. Avocado Toast on Whole Grain Bread

Ingredients:

- 1 slice whole grain bread
- 1/2 medium avocado, mashed
- 1 tsp lemon juice
- 1/4 tsp salt
- 1/8 tsp black pepper

Snacks

PreparationTime: 5 minutes
Total Time: 5 minutes
Serves: 1

↓↓

1. Toast the slice of whole grain bread.

2. In a small bowl, mash the avocado with the lemon juice, salt, and black pepper until well combined. Spread the mashed avocado mixture evenly over the toasted bread slice.

Nutritional Information (per serving):
- Calories: 250
- Total Carbs: 25g
- Fiber: 9g
- Net Carbs: 16g
- Protein: 6g
- Fat: 15g

This avocado toast on whole grain bread is an excellent snack choice for adults with type 1 diabetes. It provides a good balance of complex carbohydrates, healthy fats, and fiber to help manage blood sugar levels.

Some key benefits of this recipe for type 1 diabetes:

- Moderate in net carbs: The 16g of net carbs per serving is a reasonable amount for a snack.
- High in fiber: The 9g of fiber per serving can help slow the absorption of carbs.
- Good source of healthy fats: The avocado provides beneficial monounsaturated fats.
- Provides protein: The whole grain bread and avocado contribute a small amount of protein.
- Nutrient-dense: Avocado and whole grain bread are rich in vitamins, minerals, and antioxidants.

When choosing the whole grain bread, look for a variety that is low in added sugars and high in fiber. As always, consult with your healthcare team for personalized dietary recommendations and portion sizes.

17. Pumpkin Seeds

Ingredients:

- 1 cup raw pumpkin seeds, rinsed and dried
- 1 tbsp olive oil or melted butter
- 1 tsp salt (or to taste)
- Optional seasonings: garlic powder, onion powder, chili powder, cumin, etc.

Snacks

PreparationTime: 10 minutes
Cook Time: 20 minutes
Total Time: 30 minutes
Serves: 4

↓↓

1. Preheat oven to 325°F (165°C).

2. In a bowl, toss the rinsed and dried pumpkin seeds with the olive oil or melted butter until evenly coated.

3. Spread the seeds in a single layer on a baking sheet.

4. Sprinkle the salt and any other desired seasonings over the seeds.

5. Roast for 15-20 minutes, stirring halfway, until the seeds are lightly golden brown and crispy.

6. Allow to cool completely before serving. The seeds will continue to crisp up as they cool.

7. Store the roasted pumpkin seeds in an airtight container for up to 1 week.

Tips:
- Be sure to thoroughly dry the seeds before roasting for best crispiness.
- Adjust roasting time as needed, keeping a close eye to prevent burning.
- Try different seasoning blends to customize the flavor.

Enjoy your homemade roasted pumpkin seeds as a healthy snack!

18. Fruit and Nut Energy Balls

Ingredients:

Snacks

PreparationTime: 15 minutes
Chilling Time: 30 minutes
Total Time: 45 minutes
Serves: 12 energy balls

- 1 cup raw almonds
- 1/2 cup raw cashews
- 1/2 cup dried cranberries or chopped dates
- 1/4 cup unsweetened shredded coconut
- 2 tbsp honey or maple syrup
- 1 tsp vanilla extract
- 1/4 tsp ground cinnamon
- Pinch of salt

↓↓

1. In a food processor, pulse the almonds and cashews until they form a coarse meal, being careful not to over-process into nut butter.

2. Transfer the nut mixture to a medium bowl. Add the dried cranberries/dates, coconut, honey/maple syrup, vanilla, cinnamon, and salt. Stir until well combined.

3. Scoop the mixture by the tablespoonful and roll into small balls with your hands.

4. Place the energy balls on a parchment-lined baking sheet and refrigerate for at least 30 minutes to allow them to firm up.

5. Store the chilled energy balls in an airtight container in the refrigerator for up to 1 week.

Nutrition Information (per energy ball):
Calories: 110
Total Carbs: 9g
Fiber: 2g
Net Carbs: 7g
Protein: 3g
Fat: 7g

Tips:
- Use a mix of nuts and seeds to increase variety and nutrients.
- Adjust sweetener to taste, depending on your personal preferences and blood sugar needs.
- These energy balls make a great portable snack for adults with type 1 diabetes.

19. Roasted Chickpeas

Ingredients:

- 1 (15 oz) can chickpeas, drained and rinsed
- 1 tbsp olive oil
- 1 tsp ground cumin
- 1 tsp paprika
- 1/2 tsp garlic powder
- 1/4 tsp salt
- 1/4 tsp black pepper

Snacks

PreparationTime: 10 minutes
Cook Time: 30 minutes
Total Time: 40 minutes
Serves: 4 (about 1/2 cup per serving)

↓↓

1. Preheat oven to 400°F (200°C). Line a baking sheet with parchment paper.

2. Pat the drained and rinsed chickpeas very dry with paper towels or a clean kitchen towel. This will help them get crispy.

3. In a medium bowl, toss the chickpeas with the olive oil, cumin, paprika, garlic powder, salt, and black pepper until evenly coated.

4. Spread the seasoned chickpeas in a single layer on the prepared baking sheet.

5. Roast for 25-30 minutes, stirring halfway, until the chickpeas are crispy and golden brown.

6. Allow the roasted chickpeas to cool completely before serving. Store the roasted chickpeas in an airtight container at room temperature for up to 1 week.

Nutrition Information (per 1/2 cup serving):
Calories: 130
Total Carbs: 18g
Fiber: 5g
Net Carbs: 13g
Protein: 6g
Fat: 4g

Tips:
- Adjust seasoning amounts to your taste preferences.
- Try different spice blends like chili powder, curry powder, or cajun seasoning.
- Roast the chickpeas in batches if needed to ensure they get crispy.
- These make a great high-fiber, high-protein snack for adults with type 1 diabetes.

20. Sliced Turkey with Cheese Roll-Ups

Ingredients:

- 8 slices deli-style turkey breast
- 4 slices cheddar or Swiss cheese
- 1 tbsp Dijon mustard (optional)

Snacks

PreparationTime: 10 minutes
Serves: 4 (2 roll-ups per serving)

↓↓

1. Lay the turkey slices out flat on a clean work surface.

2. Place a slice of cheese on each turkey slice.

3. If using, spread a thin layer of Dijon mustard over the cheese.

4. Carefully roll up each turkey and cheese slice into a tight cylinder.

5. Secure the roll-ups with toothpicks or cut them in half to serve.

Nutrition Information (per 2 roll-up serving):
Calories: 150
Total Carbs: 1g
Fiber: 0g
Net Carbs: 1g
Protein: 16g
Fat: 9g

Tips:
- Choose low-sodium turkey and reduced-fat cheese to keep sodium and saturated fat in check.
- Experiment with different cheese varieties like pepper jack or provolone.
- Add a thin slice of dill pickle or a smear of cream cheese for extra flavor.
- These roll-ups make a quick, portable, and protein-rich snack or light meal for adults with type 1 diabetes.
- Pair with fresh veggies, nuts, or a small side salad for a more complete meal.

1. Berry Chia Seed Jam

Ingredients:

- 2 cups fresh or frozen mixed berries
 (such as raspberries, blackberries, blueberries)
- 2 tbsp chia seeds
- 1-2 tbsp honey or maple syrup (to taste)
- 1 tsp lemon juice

Desserts

PreparationTime: 10 minutes
Cook Time: 10 minutes
Total Time: 20 minutes
Serves: 8 (2 tbsp per serving)

↓↓↓

1. In a medium saucepan, combine the berries, chia seeds, 1 tbsp of honey/maple syrup, and lemon juice.

2. Cook over medium heat, stirring frequently, until the berries break down and the mixture thickens, about 8-10 minutes.

3. Taste and add an additional 1 tbsp of honey/maple syrup if desired, for a sweeter jam.

4. Remove from heat and let cool slightly. The jam will continue to thicken as it cools.

5. Transfer the jam to a clean jar or airtight container and refrigerate for up to 1 week.

Nutrition Information (per 2 tbsp serving):
Calories: 50
Total Carbs: 8g
Fiber: 3g
Net Carbs: 5g
Protein: 1g
Fat: 2g

Tips:
- Use a mix of berries for more flavor and nutrients.
- Adjust sweetener to your taste preferences and blood sugar needs.
- Chia seeds provide fiber, protein, and healthy omega-3 fatty acids.
- Enjoy the jam on whole grain toast, crackers, or as a topping for Greek yogurt or oatmeal.
- This homemade jam is a healthier alternative to store-bought options for adults with type 1 diabetes.

2. Greek Yogurt with a Drizzle of Honey

Ingredients:

- 1 cup plain Greek yogurt
- 1-2 tsp honey (to taste)

Desserts

PreparationTime: 5 minutes
Serves: 1

↓↓

1. Scoop the Greek yogurt into a serving bowl or container.

2. Drizzle the honey over the top of the yogurt.

3. Gently stir the honey into the yogurt until well combined.

Nutrition Information:
- 1 cup plain Greek yogurt:
  - Calories: 140
  - Total Carbs: 6g
  - Fiber: 0g
  - Net Carbs: 6g
  - Protein: 23g
  - Fat: 4g
- 1 tsp honey:
  - Calories: 22
  - Total Carbs: 6g
  - Fiber: 0g
  - Net Carbs: 6g
  - Protein: 0g
  - Fat: 0g

Total Nutrition Information (with 1 tsp honey):
Calories: 162 Total Carbs: 12g Fiber: 0g Net Carbs: 12g Protein: 23g Fat: 4g

Tips:
- Use 1-2 tsp of honey, depending on your personal taste preferences and blood sugar needs.
- Greek yogurt is high in protein and low in carbs, making it a great choice for adults with type 1 diabetes.
- Top with fresh berries, nuts, or a sprinkle of cinnamon for added flavor and nutrition.
- This simple snack or light meal provides a balance of protein, carbs, and healthy fats.

3. Almond Flour Brownies

Ingredients:

- 1 cup (100g) almond flour
- 1/4 cup (30g) unsweetened cocoa powder
- 1/4 tsp salt
- 1/2 cup (120ml) melted coconut oil or unsalted butter
- 1/2 cup (120ml) granulated erythritol or Swerve
- 2 large eggs
- 1 tsp vanilla extract

Desserts

PreparationTime: 15 minutes
Cook Time: 25 minutes
Total Time: 40 minutes
Serves: 16 brownies

↓↓

1. Preheat oven to 350°F (175°C). Grease an 8x8 inch baking pan.

2. In a medium bowl, whisk together the almond flour, cocoa powder, and salt.

3. In a separate bowl, beat together the melted coconut oil/butter, erythritol/Swerve, eggs, and vanilla until well combined.

4. Gradually stir the wet ingredients into the dry ingredients until a thick batter forms.

5. Spread the batter evenly into the prepared baking pan.

6. Bake for 22-25 minutes, until a toothpick inserted in the center comes out clean.

7. Allow the brownies to cool completely in the pan before cutting into 16 squares.

Nutrition Information (per brownie):
Calories: 110 - Total Carbs: 4g
Fiber: 2g - Net Carbs: 2g - Protein: 3g - Fat: 10g

Tips:
- Use a sugar-free granulated sweetener like erythritol or Swerve to keep the carbs low.
- Almond flour provides a moist, fudgy texture without the need for regular flour.
- Store the brownies in an airtight container at room temperature for up to 5 days.
- Enjoy these low-carb, high-fat brownies as an occasional treat for adults with type 1 diabetes.

4. Baked Apples with Cinnamon

Ingredients:

- 4 medium apples, cored and halved
- 2 tbsp unsalted butter, melted
- 2 tbsp granulated erythritol or Swerve
- 1 tsp ground cinnamon
- 1/4 tsp ground nutmeg (optional)
- 2 tbsp chopped walnuts or pecans (optional)

Desserts

PreparationTime: 10 minutes
Cook Time: 30 minutes
Total Time: 40 minutes
Serves: 4

↓↓

1. Preheat oven to 375°F (190°C). Grease a baking dish or line with parchment paper.

2. Place the apple halves cut-side up in the prepared baking dish.

3. In a small bowl, mix together the melted butter, erythritol/Swerve, cinnamon, and nutmeg (if using).

4. Spoon the cinnamon-butter mixture evenly over the top of the apple halves.

5. Bake for 25-30 minutes, until the apples are tender when pierced with a fork.

6. Remove from oven and sprinkle the chopped nuts over the top, if using.

7. Serve the baked apples warm.

Nutrition Information (per serving, without nuts):
Calories: 100
Total Carbs: 15g
Fiber: 3g
Net Carbs: 12g
Protein: 0g
Fat: 5g

Tips:
- Use a sugar-free granulated sweetener like erythritol or Swerve to keep the carbs low.
- Choose firm, tart apples like Granny Smith or Honeycrisp for best results.
- Add a dollop of unsweetened whipped cream or a scoop of vanilla Greek yogurt for extra creaminess.
- These baked apples make a delicious, low-carb dessert or snack for adults with type 1 diabetes.

5. Coconut Milk Ice Cream

Ingredients:

- 1 (13.5 oz) can full-fat coconut milk
- 1/4 cup granulated erythritol or Swerve
- 1 tsp vanilla extract
- 1/4 tsp xanthan gum (optional, for creamier texture)

Desserts

PreparationTime: 10 minutes
Chilling Time: 4-6 hours
Total Time: 4-6 hours 10 minutes
Serves: 4 (1/2 cup per serving)

↓↓

1. In a medium bowl, whisk together the coconut milk, erythritol/Swerve, vanilla, and xanthan gum (if using) until well combined.

2. Pour the mixture into a shallow baking dish or metal pan and place in the freezer.

3. After 45 minutes, remove the pan from the freezer and stir the mixture with a fork to break up any ice crystals that have formed.

4. Return the pan to the freezer and repeat the stirring process every 45 minutes for 3-4 hours, until the ice cream reaches your desired consistency.

5. Once the ice cream has reached a scoopable texture, transfer it to an airtight container and freeze for an additional 1-2 hours before serving.

Nutrition Information (per 1/2 cup serving):
Calories: 160
Total Carbs: 5g
Fiber: 1g
Net Carbs: 4g
Protein: 1g
Fat: 15g

Tips:
- Use a sugar-free granulated sweetener like erythritol or Swerve to keep the carbs low.
- The xanthan gum is optional, but it can help create a creamier, smoother texture.
- Experiment with different flavor additions, such as unsweetened cocoa powder, cinnamon, or chopped nuts.
- Store the homemade ice cream in the freezer for up to 2 weeks.
- This coconut milk-based ice cream is a delicious, low-carb treat for adults with type 1 diabetes.

6. Chocolate Avocado Mousse

Ingredients:

- 2 ripe avocados, pitted and flesh scooped out
- 1/4 cup unsweetened cocoa powder
- 1/4 cup granulated erythritol or Swerve
- 1/4 cup unsweetened almond milk
- 1 tsp vanilla extract
- 1/4 tsp sea salt

Desserts

PreparationTime: 10 minutes
Chilling Time: 2 hours
Total Time: 2 hours 10 minutes
Serves: 4 (1/2 cup per serving)

↓↓

1. In a food processor or high-powered blender, combine the avocado flesh, cocoa powder, erythritol/Swerve, almond milk, vanilla, and salt. Blend until smooth and creamy, scraping down the sides as needed.

2. Divide the chocolate avocado mousse evenly into 4 small ramekins or serving dishes.

3. Cover and refrigerate for at least 2 hours, or until set.

4. Serve chilled, garnished with a sprinkle of cocoa powder, chopped nuts, or fresh berries if desired.

Nutrition Information (per 1/2 cup serving):
Calories: 170
Total Carbs: 10g
Fiber: 7g
Net Carbs: 3g
Protein: 3g
Fat: 15g

Tips:
- Use a sugar-free granulated sweetener like erythritol or Swerve to keep the carbs low.
- Ripe avocados provide a rich, creamy texture without the need for heavy cream or dairy.
- Adjust the amount of sweetener to your personal taste preferences.
- This mousse can be made ahead of time and stored in the refrigerator for up to 3 days.
- Enjoy this decadent, low-carb chocolate treat as a healthy dessert or snack.

7. Mixed Berry Sorbet

Ingredients:

- 2 cups mixed berries
 (such as raspberries, blackberries, blueberries)
- 1/4 cup granulated erythritol or Swerve
- 1 tbsp fresh lemon juice

Desserts

PreparationTime: 10 minutes
Freezing Time: 4-6 hours
Total Time: 4-6 hours 10 minutes
Serves: 4 (1/2 cup per serving)

↓↓

1. In a food processor or high-powered blender, combine the mixed berries, erythritol/Swerve, and lemon juice. Blend until smooth.

2. Pour the berry mixture into a shallow baking dish or metal pan and place in the freezer.

3. After 45 minutes, remove the pan from the freezer and stir the mixture with a fork to break up any ice crystals that have formed.

4. Return the pan to the freezer and repeat the stirring process every 45 minutes for 3-4 hours, until the sorbet reaches your desired consistency.

5. Once the sorbet has reached a scoopable texture, transfer it to an airtight container and freeze for an additional 1-2 hours before serving.

Nutrition Information (per 1/2 cup serving):
Calories: 50
Total Carbs: 10g
Fiber: 3g
Net Carbs: 7g
Protein: 1g
Fat: 0g

Tips:
- Use a sugar-free granulated sweetener like erythritol or Swerve to keep the carbs low.
- Adjust the amount of sweetener to your personal taste preferences.
- Experiment with different berry combinations, such as strawberry-kiwi or mango-pineapple.
- Serve the sorbet in small portions, as it can be quite sweet.
- Store the homemade sorbet in the freezer for up to 2 weeks.
- This refreshing, low-carb sorbet makes a great palate-cleansing dessert or snack.

8. Nut and Seed Granola Bars

Ingredients:

Desserts

- 1 cup raw almonds, chopped
- 1/2 cup raw pumpkin seeds
- 1/2 cup raw sunflower seeds
- 1/2 cup unsweetened shredded coconut
- 1/4 cup ground flaxseed
- 1/4 cup chia seeds
- 1/4 cup unsweetened almond butter
- 1/4 cup honey or maple syrup
- 1 tsp vanilla extract
- 1/4 tsp sea salt

PreparationTime: 15 minutes
Bake Time: 20 minutes
Cooling Time: 30 minutes
Total Time: 1 hour 5 minutes
Serves: 12 bars

↓↓↓

1. Preheat oven to 325°F (165°C). Line an 8x8 inch baking pan with parchment paper, leaving some overhang on the sides.

2. In a large bowl, combine the chopped almonds, pumpkin seeds, sunflower seeds, shredded coconut, ground flaxseed, and chia seeds. Mix well.

3. In a small saucepan, heat the almond butter and honey/maple syrup over low heat, stirring constantly, until smooth and combined.

4. Remove the almond butter mixture from heat and stir in the vanilla and salt.

5. Pour the almond butter mixture over the dry ingredients and stir until well coated.

6. Press the granola bar mixture firmly into the prepared baking pan, using a spatula or your hands to compact it.

7. Bake for 18-20 minutes, until lightly golden.

8. Allow the granola bars to cool completely in the pan, about 30 minutes.

9. Lift the bars out of the pan using the parchment paper overhang and cut into 12 bars.

Nutrition Information (per bar):
Calories: 180 - Total Carbs: 12g - Fiber: 4g - Net Carbs: 8g - Protein: 5g - Fat: 13g

Tips:
- Use a sugar-free liquid sweetener like monk fruit syrup or sugar-free maple syrup to reduce the carbs.
- Customize the nuts and seeds to your preference, but maintain the overall ratio.
- Store the granola bars in an airtight container at room temperature for up to 1 week.
- These nutrient-dense bars make a great portable snack or breakfast option.

9. Pumpkin Pie with Almond Crust

Ingredients:

- 1 1/2 cups almond flour
- 2 tbsp granulated erythritol or Swerve
- 3 tbsp unsalted butter, melted
- 1/4 tsp ground cinnamon

Filling Ingredients:
- 1 (15 oz) can pumpkin puree
- 3 large eggs
- 1/2 cup unsweetened almond milk
- 1/2 cup granulated erythritol or Swerve
- 1 tsp ground cinnamon
- 1/2 tsp ground ginger
- 1/4 tsp ground nutmeg
- 1/4 tsp ground cloves
- 1/4 tsp salt

↓↓↓

Crust:
1. Preheat oven to 350°F (175°C). Grease a 9-inch pie dish.
2. In a medium bowl, mix together the almond flour, erythritol/Swerve, melted butter, and cinnamon until well combined.
3. Press the mixture evenly into the bottom and up the sides of the prepared pie dish.
4. Bake for 10-12 minutes, then let cool completely.

Filling:
1. In a large bowl, whisk together the pumpkin puree, eggs, almond milk, erythritol/Swerve, cinnamon, ginger, nutmeg, cloves, and salt until smooth.
2. Pour the filling into the prepared almond flour crust.
3. Bake for 40-45 minutes, until the center is almost set.
4. Allow the pie to cool completely, then refrigerate for at least 2 hours before serving.

Nutrition Information (per slice):
Calories: 220 - Total Carbs: 12g - Fiber: 3g - Net Carbs: 9g - Protein: 6g Fat: 18g

Tips:
- Use a sugar-free granulated sweetener like erythritol or Swerve to keep the carbs low.
- The almond flour crust provides a delicious, nutty base for the pumpkin filling.
- Serve with a dollop of unsweetened whipped cream or a sprinkle of cinnamon, if desired.

10. Sugar-Free Jello with Fresh Fruit

Ingredients:

- 1 (3 oz) package sugar-free Jello (any flavor)
- 1 cup boiling water
- 1 cup cold water
- 1 cup mixed fresh fruit (such as berries, melon, kiwi)

↓↓

1. In a medium bowl, dissolve the Jello powder in the boiling water, stirring for 2-3 minutes until completely dissolved.

2. Add the cold water and stir to combine.

3. Refrigerate the Jello mixture for 30-45 minutes, or until it starts to thicken slightly.

4. Gently fold in the mixed fresh fruit.

5. Pour the Jello and fruit mixture into individual serving dishes or a larger serving bowl.

6. Refrigerate for at least 2 hours, or until the Jello is fully set.

Nutrition Information (per 1/2 cup serving):
- Sugar-Free Jello (any flavor):
  - Calories: 10   - Total Carbs: 2g   - Fiber: 0g - Net Carbs: 2g - Protein: 0g - Fat: 0g
- 1/2 cup mixed fresh fruit:
  - Calories: 30-50
  - Total Carbs: 7-12g
  - Fiber: 1-3g
  - Net Carbs: 6-9g
  - Protein: 0-1g
  - Fat: 0g

Total Nutrition Information (per 1/2 cup serving):
Calories: 40-60 Total Carbs: 9-14g- Fiber: 1-3g - Net Carbs: 8-11g = Protein: 0-1g
Fat: 0g

Tips:
- Choose sugar-free Jello flavors that you enjoy, such as strawberry, raspberry, or lemon.
- Opt for a variety of fresh, low-glycemic fruits like berries, melon, and kiwi.
- Adjust the amount of fruit to your personal taste and carb preferences.
- This refreshing, low-carb dessert is a great option for adults with type 1 diabetes.

11. Baked Pears with Walnuts

Ingredients:

- 4 ripe but firm pears, halved and cored
- 2 tbsp unsalted butter, melted
- 2 tbsp granulated erythritol or Swerve
- 1/4 cup chopped walnuts
- 1 tsp ground cinnamon

Desserts

PreparationTime: 10 minutes
Cook Time: 30 minutes
Total Time: 40 minutes
Serves: 4

↓↓↓

1. Preheat oven to 375°F (190°C). Grease a baking dish or line with parchment paper.

2. Place the pear halves cut-side up in the prepared baking dish.

3. In a small bowl, mix together the melted butter, erythritol/Swerve, and cinnamon.

4. Spoon the butter-sweetener mixture evenly over the top of the pear halves.

5. Sprinkle the chopped walnuts over the pears.

6. Bake for 25-30 minutes, or until the pears are tender when pierced with a fork.

7. Serve the baked pears warm, with the juices from the baking dish spooned over the top.

Nutrition Information (per serving):
Calories: 160 - Total Carbs: 18g
Fiber: 4g - Net Carbs: 14g - Protein: 2g - Fat: 9g

Tips:
- Use a sugar-free granulated sweetener like erythritol or Swerve to keep the carbs low.
- Choose firm, ripe pears that will hold their shape during baking.
- Adjust the amount of sweetener to your personal taste preferences and blood sugar needs.
- Serve the baked pears with a dollop of unsweetened whipped cream or a sprinkle of chopped nuts for added texture and flavor.
- This warm, comforting dessert is a great option for adults with type 1 diabetes.

12. Low-Carb Cheesecake Bites

Ingredients:

- 1 cup almond flour
- 2 tbsp granulated erythritol or Swerve
- 3 tbsp unsalted butter, melted

Filling Ingredients:
- 8 oz cream cheese, softened
- 1/4 cup granulated erythritol or Swerve
- 1 tsp vanilla extract
- 1 large egg
- 1/4 cup heavy cream

Desserts

PreparationTime: 15 minutes
Chilling Time: 2 hours
Total Time: 2 hours 15 minutes
Serves: 12 bites

Crust

↓↓

Crust:
1. Line a 12-cup mini muffin tin with paper liners.
2. In a small bowl, mix together the almond flour, erythritol/Swerve, and melted butter until well combined.
3. Divide the crust mixture evenly among the muffin cups, pressing it into the bottom and slightly up the sides.

Filling:
1. In a medium bowl, beat the cream cheese with an electric mixer until smooth and creamy.
2. Add the erythritol/Swerve, vanilla, egg, and heavy cream. Beat until well combined and the mixture is light and fluffy.
3. Spoon the cheesecake filling evenly over the crust in the muffin cups.
4. Refrigerate the cheesecake bites for at least 2 hours, or until set.

Nutrition Information (per bite):
Calories: 130 - Total Carbs: 3g - Fiber: 1g - Net Carbs: 2g - Protein: 3g - Fat: 12g

Tips:
- Use a sugar-free granulated sweetener like erythritol or Swerve to keep the carbs low.
- Adjust the amount of sweetener to your personal taste preferences.
- Top the chilled cheesecake bites with a fresh raspberry or a sprinkle of cinnamon, if desired.
- Store the cheesecake bites in the refrigerator for up to 5 days.
- These low-carb, portion-controlled cheesecake bites make a great dessert or snack for adults with type 1 diabetes.

13. Cinnamon-Spiced Almonds

Ingredients:

- 2 cups raw almonds
- 1 tbsp granulated erythritol or Swerve
- 1 tsp ground cinnamon
- 1/4 tsp ground nutmeg
- 1/4 tsp sea salt

Desserts

PreparationTime: 5 minutes
Cook Time: 15 minutes
Total Time: 20 minutes
Serves: 8 (1/4 cup per serving)

↓↓

1. Preheat oven to 325°F (165°C). Line a baking sheet with parchment paper.

2. In a medium bowl, toss the raw almonds with the erythritol/Swerve, cinnamon, nutmeg, and salt until the almonds are evenly coated.

3. Spread the seasoned almonds in a single layer on the prepared baking sheet.

4. Bake for 12-15 minutes, stirring halfway, until the almonds are fragrant and lightly toasted.

5. Allow the cinnamon-spiced almonds to cool completely on the baking sheet before serving.

6. Store the cooled almonds in an airtight container at room temperature for up to 1 week.

Nutrition Information (per 1/4 cup serving):
Calories: 160 - Total Carbs: 5g - Fiber: 3g
Net Carbs: 2g - Protein: 6gFat: 14g

Tips:
- Use a sugar-free granulated sweetener like erythritol or Swerve to keep the carbs low.
- Adjust the amount of sweetener and spices to your personal taste preferences.
- Try adding a pinch of cayenne pepper for a touch of heat.
- These cinnamon-spiced almonds make a great portable, low-carb snack for adults with type 1 diabetes.
- Pair them with fresh berries or a small piece of dark chocolate for a more satisfying treat.

14. Chocolate-Dipped Strawberries

Ingredients:

- 12 fresh strawberries, washed and patted dry
- 2 oz sugar-free dark chocolate, chopped
- 1 tsp coconut oil

Desserts

PreparationTime: 15 minutes
Chilling Time: 30 minutes
Total Time: 45 minutes
Serves: 12 strawberries (1 strawberry per serving)

1. Line a baking sheet with parchment paper.

2. In a small microwave-safe bowl, combine the chopped sugar-free dark chocolate and coconut oil. Microwave in 30-second intervals, stirring between each, until the chocolate is melted and smooth.

3. Holding them by the stem, dip each strawberry into the melted chocolate, coating about three-quarters of the berry.

4. Place the chocolate-dipped strawberries on the prepared baking sheet and refrigerate for at least 30 minutes, or until the chocolate has hardened.

Nutrition Information (per strawberry):
Calories: 35
Total Carbs: 4g
Fiber: 1g
Net Carbs: 3g
Protein: 1g
Fat: 2g

Tips:
- Use a high-quality, sugar-free dark chocolate with a minimum of 70% cacao content.
- The coconut oil helps the chocolate harden and creates a nice sheen.
- Refrigerate the chocolate-dipped strawberries until ready to serve for the best texture.
- These make a delightful, low-carb treat for adults with type 1 diabetes.
- Enjoy the strawberries as a standalone dessert or pair them with a small serving of unsweetened whipped cream.

15. Frozen Yogurt Bark with Nuts and Seeds

Ingredients:

- 2 cups plain Greek yogurt
- 2 tbsp granulated erythritol or Swerve
- 1 tsp vanilla extract
- 1/4 cup chopped walnuts
- 2 tbsp unsweetened shredded coconut
- 2 tbsp chia seeds
- 2 tbsp pumpkin seeds

Desserts

PreparationTime: 10 minutes
Freezing Time: 2-3 hours
Total Time: 2-3 hours 10 minutes
Serves: 8 (1/2 cup per serving)

↓↓↓

1. Line a baking sheet with parchment paper.

2. In a medium bowl, mix together the Greek yogurt, erythritol/Swerve, and vanilla until well combined.

3. Spread the yogurt mixture evenly onto the prepared baking sheet, creating a rectangular shape about 1/4 inch thick.

4. Sprinkle the chopped walnuts, shredded coconut, chia seeds, and pumpkin seeds evenly over the top of the yogurt.

5. Freeze for 2-3 hours, or until the yogurt bark is completely frozen.

6. Break or cut the frozen yogurt bark into 8 pieces and serve immediately.

7. Store any leftover pieces in an airtight container in the freezer for up to 1 month.

Nutrition Information (per 1/2 cup serving):
Calories: 130 - Total Carbs: 8g - Fiber: 3g - Net Carbs: 5g - Protein: 10g - Fat: 8g

Tips:
- Use a sugar-free granulated sweetener like erythritol or Swerve to keep the carbs low.
- Adjust the amount of sweetener to your personal taste preferences.
- Customize the nuts and seeds based on your preferences and what you have on hand.
- This frozen yogurt bark makes a refreshing, protein-packed snack or dessert for adults with type 1 diabetes.

16. Coconut Macaroons

Ingredients:

- 2 cups unsweetened shredded coconut
- 1/4 cup granulated erythritol or Swerve
- 2 large egg whites
- 1 tsp vanilla extract
- 1/8 tsp salt

PreparationTime: 10 minutes
Bake Time: 12-15 minutes
Total Time: 22-25 minutes
Serves: 12 macaroons

↓↓

1. Preheat oven to 325°F (165°C). Line a baking sheet with parchment paper.

2. In a medium bowl, mix together the shredded coconut and erythritol/Swerve.

3. In a separate small bowl, beat the egg whites until they are foamy and hold soft peaks.

4. Gently fold the beaten egg whites, vanilla, and salt into the coconut mixture until well combined.

5. Scoop the coconut mixture by the tablespoonful and place the mounds onto the prepared baking sheet, spacing them about 1 inch apart.

6. Bake for 12-15 minutes, or until the macaroons are lightly golden brown on the edges.

7. Allow the macaroons to cool on the baking sheet for 5 minutes before transferring them to a wire rack to cool completely.

Nutrition Information (per macaroon):
Calories: 70 = Total Carbs: 4g - Fiber: 2g - Net Carbs: 2g Protein: 1g
Fat: 6g

Tips:
- Use a sugar-free granulated sweetener like erythritol or Swerve to keep the carbs low.
- Adjust the amount of sweetener to your personal taste preferences.
- For a chewier texture, bake the macaroons for the shorter end of the time range.
- Store the cooled macaroons in an airtight container at room temperature for up to 1 week.
- These coconut macaroons make a delightful, low-carb treat for adults with type 1 diabetes.

17. Almond Butter Cookies

Ingredients:

- 1 cup creamy unsweetened almond butter
- 1/2 cup granulated erythritol or Swerve
- 1 large egg
- 1 tsp vanilla extract
- 1/4 tsp sea salt

Desserts

PreparationTime: 10 minutes
Bake Time: 10-12 minutes
Total Time: 20-22 minutes
Serves: 12 cookies

↓↓

1. Preheat oven to 350°F (175°C). Line a baking sheet with parchment paper.

2. In a medium bowl, mix together the almond butter, erythritol/Swerve, egg, vanilla, and salt until well combined.

3. Scoop the dough by the tablespoonful and roll into balls. Place the balls about 2 inches apart on the prepared baking sheet.

4. Use a fork to gently press down on each cookie, creating a criss-cross pattern.

5. Bake for 10-12 minutes, or until the cookies are lightly golden around the edges.

6. Allow the cookies to cool on the baking sheet for 5 minutes before transferring them to a wire rack to cool completely.

Nutrition Information (per cookie):
Calories: 100
Total Carbs: 3g
Fiber: 1g
Net Carbs: 2g
Protein: 3g
Fat: 9g

Tips:
- Use a sugar-free granulated sweetener like erythritol or Swerve to keep the carbs low.
- Adjust the amount of sweetener to your personal taste preferences.
- For a chunkier texture, use crunchy almond butter instead of creamy.
- Store the cooled cookies in an airtight container at room temperature for up to 1 week.
- These almond butter cookies make a delicious, low-carb snack or dessert for adults with type 1 diabetes.

18. Ricotta Cheese with Berries

Ingredients:

- 1/2 cup full-fat ricotta cheese
- 1/2 cup mixed fresh berries
 (such as raspberries, blackberries, blueberries)
- 1 tsp granulated erythritol or Swerve (optional)

Desserts

PreparationTime: 5 minutes
Serves: 1

↓↓

1. Scoop the ricotta cheese into a small bowl or serving dish.

2. Top the ricotta with the mixed fresh berries.

3. If desired, sprinkle the erythritol/Swerve over the top of the berries to add a light sweetness.

Nutrition Information (without sweetener):
Calories: 220
Total Carbs: 10g
Fiber: 3g
Net Carbs: 7g
Protein: 15g
Fat: 13g

Tips:
- Use full-fat ricotta cheese for a richer, creamier texture.
- Choose a variety of fresh, low-glycemic berries for added nutrients and flavor.
- Add the sweetener only if needed, as the berries provide natural sweetness.
- This simple, protein-packed snack or light meal is a great option for adults with type 1 diabetes.
- Pair it with a small handful of nuts or a few slices of cucumber for a more complete and satisfying dish.
- Adjust the portion sizes as needed to fit your individual carb and calorie needs.

19. Baked Cinnamon Apples with a Crumb Topping

Ingredients:

- 4 medium apples, peeled, cored, and sliced
- 2 tbsp granulated erythritol or Swerve
- 1 tsp ground cinnamon
- 1/4 tsp ground nutmeg

Crumb Topping Ingredients:
- 1/2 cup almond flour
- 2 tbsp granulated erythritol or Swerve
- 2 tbsp unsalted butter, melted
- 1/2 tsp ground cinnamon

Desserts

PreparationTime: 15 minutes
Bake Time: 30 minutes
Total Time: 45 minutes
Serves: 4

Filling

↓↓

1. Preheat oven to 375°F (190°C). Grease a baking dish.

Filling:
2. In a large bowl, toss the sliced apples with the erythritol/Swerve, cinnamon, and nutmeg until well coated.
3. Transfer the apple mixture to the prepared baking dish.

Crumb Topping:
4. In a small bowl, mix together the almond flour, erythritol/Swerve, melted butter, and cinnamon until a crumbly mixture forms.
5. Sprinkle the crumb topping evenly over the apple filling.

Baking:
6. Bake for 30 minutes, or until the apples are tender and the topping is lightly golden.
7. Allow the baked apples to cool for 5-10 minutes before serving.

Nutrition Information (per serving):
Calories: 180 - Total Carbs: 18g - Fiber: 4g - Net Carbs: 14g
Protein: 2g - Fat: 10g

Tips:
- Use a sugar-free granulated sweetener like erythritol or Swerve to keep the carbs low.
- Adjust the amount of sweetener to your personal taste preferences.
- Serve the baked cinnamon apples warm, with a dollop of unsweetened whipped cream or a sprinkle of chopped nuts, if desired.
- This comforting, low-carb dessert is a great option for adults with type 1 diabetes.

20. Diabetic-Friendly Fruit Salad

Ingredients:

Desserts

PreparationTime: 15 minutes
Serves: 4 (1 cup per serving)

- 1 cup diced watermelon
- 1 cup diced cantaloupe
- 1 cup blueberries
- 1 cup raspberries
- 2 tbsp fresh lemon juice
- 1 tbsp granulated erythritol or Swerve (optional)

↓↓↓

1. In a large bowl, combine the diced watermelon, cantaloupe, blueberries, and raspberries.

2. Drizzle the fresh lemon juice over the fruit and gently toss to coat.

3. If desired, sprinkle the erythritol/Swerve over the fruit salad and toss again to distribute the sweetener.

Nutrition Information (per 1 cup serving, without sweetener):
Calories: 80
Total Carbs: 18g
Fiber: 4g
Net Carbs: 14g
Protein: 1g
Fat: 0g

Tips:
- Choose a variety of low-glycemic fruits like berries, melon, and citrus.
- Adjust the amount of sweetener to your personal taste preferences and blood sugar needs.
- Serve the fruit salad chilled for a refreshing and hydrating snack or light dessert.
- This diabetic-friendly fruit salad is a great way to incorporate more fiber, vitamins, and antioxidants into your diet.
- Pair it with a small serving of plain Greek yogurt or a handful of nuts for a more balanced snack.

Meal Planning and Preparation

Effective meal planning and preparation are key to managing type 1 diabetes and maintaining balanced blood sugar levels. By organizing your meals and snacks in advance, you can ensure that you're consuming nutritious foods that align with your diabetes management goals. This section will provide practical tips for meal planning, shopping, and preparation to make your journey easier and more enjoyable.

Tips for Effective Meal Planning

- **Create a Weekly Meal Plan**
  - Plan Ahead: Set aside time each week to plan your meals. This will help you make informed choices and avoid last-minute decisions that could lead to less healthy options.

  - Balance Your Meals: Include a variety of food groups in each meal, such as lean proteins, whole grains, healthy fats, and plenty of vegetables. This ensures a balanced intake of nutrients and helps keep blood sugar levels stable.

  - Portion Control: Pay attention to portion sizes to manage carbohydrate intake and prevent overeating. Use measuring cups or a kitchen scale if needed to keep portions consistent.

- **Incorporate a Variety of Recipes**
  - Mix It Up: Rotate recipes to keep meals interesting and prevent boredom. This also helps ensure that you're getting a wide range of nutrients.

  - Adapt Recipes: Modify recipes to suit your taste preferences and dietary needs. For example, you can adjust ingredient quantities or substitute ingredients to meet your nutritional goals.

- **Prepare Ahead**
  - Batch Cooking: Cook larger quantities of meals and freeze individual portions for quick and convenient options on busy days. This can save time and reduce the temptation to choose less healthy options.
  -
  - Pre-Chop Vegetables: Wash and chop vegetables in advance and store them in airtight containers in the refrigerator. This makes meal preparation faster and easier.

- **Use a Meal Planning Tool**
  - Apps and Tools: Consider using meal planning apps or tools to organize your recipes, create shopping lists, and track your nutritional intake. These tools can help simplify the planning process and keep you on track.

Shopping Lists and Pantry Staples

- Create a Shopping List
  - Plan Your List: Based on your meal plan, create a detailed shopping list to ensure you have all the ingredients you need. This helps avoid impulse purchases and ensures you have the right foods on hand.

  - Stick to Your List: When shopping, stick to your list to avoid buying items that might not fit into your meal plan or could negatively impact your blood sugar levels.

- Stock Your Pantry
  - Healthy Staples: Keep your pantry stocked with diabetes-friendly staples, such as whole grains, canned beans, low-sodium vegetables, and nuts. These items can be used to create quick and nutritious meals.

  - Low-Carb Options: Include low-carb options like almond flour, chia seeds, and non-starchy vegetables to help manage carbohydrate intake.

Cooking and Portion Control
- Cooking Techniques
  - Healthy Cooking Methods: Opt for healthy cooking methods such as grilling, baking, steaming, or sautéing with minimal oil. Avoid frying or using excessive amounts of butter or oil.

  - Flavor Without Extra Carbs: Use herbs, spices, and citrus to add flavor to your dishes without adding extra carbohydrates or sodium.
- Portion Control

  - Use Portion Control Tools: Invest in portion control tools like measuring cups and food scales to help manage portion sizes accurately.
  - Plate Your Meals: Use smaller plates to help control portion sizes and prevent overeating. Aim to fill half your plate with vegetables, a quarter with lean protein, and a quarter with whole grains or starchy vegetables.

- Monitor Blood Sugar Levels
  - Adjust as Needed: Pay attention to how different foods affect your blood sugar levels and adjust your meal plan accordingly. Keep track of your blood sugar readings and consult with your healthcare provider to make any necessary adjustments.

By implementing these meal planning and preparation strategies, you can make managing type 1 diabetes more manageable and less stressful. Consistent planning and preparation not only support better blood sugar control but also contribute to overall well-being. Enjoy the process of creating delicious, balanced meals that support your health goals!

Nutritional Information

Understanding nutritional information is crucial for managing type 1 diabetes effectively. This section will help you interpret nutrition labels, calculate carbohydrates, and make informed food choices to maintain stable blood sugar levels and support overall health.

Understanding Nutritional Labels

- Serving Size
  - Definition: The serving size listed on a nutrition label is the amount that the nutritional information refers to. It's important to compare this with the portion size you consume to accurately assess the nutritional content.

  - Tip: Measure your portions to ensure they match the serving size listed on the label, especially if you're trying to manage carbohydrate intake.

- Calories
  - Definition: Calories measure the amount of energy provided by a food. While not directly related to blood sugar, managing calorie intake is important for overall health and weight management.

  - Tip: Focus on nutrient-dense foods that provide essential vitamins and minerals without excessive calories.

- Total Carbohydrates
  - Definition: This includes all carbohydrates in the food, such as sugars, starches, and fiber. Carbohydrates have the most significant impact on blood sugar levels.

  - Tip: Pay attention to the total carbohydrate content and how it fits into your daily carbohydrate goals. Use a carbohydrate counting method or a diabetes management app to track your intake.
- Fiber

  - Definition: Fiber is a type of carbohydrate that is not digested by the body. It can help regulate blood sugar levels and support digestive health.

  - Tip: Foods high in fiber can help stabilize blood sugar levels. Aim for high-fiber foods, such as vegetables, fruits, and whole grains.

- Sugars

  - Definition: This includes both natural and added sugars. Added sugars can cause rapid spikes in blood glucose levels.

- Tip: Limit foods with high amounts of added sugars. Opt for naturally sweet foods like fruits and use them in moderation.

- Protein

  - Definition: Protein helps maintain muscle mass and supports overall health. It also has a minimal impact on blood sugar levels.

  - Tip: Include lean protein sources in your meals, such as poultry, fish, beans, and tofu.

- Fats
  - Types:

    - Total Fat: Indicates the total amount of fat in the food. Fats are essential for health but should be consumed in moderation.

    - Saturated Fat: Consuming high amounts can increase the risk of heart disease. Choose foods low in saturated fat.

    - Trans Fat: These are unhealthy fats that should be avoided as much as possible.

    - Unsaturated Fat: Healthy fats found in sources like avocados, nuts, and olive oil.

  - Tip: Focus on healthy fats and limit saturated and trans fats to support cardiovascular health.

- Sodium

  - Definition: Sodium is a mineral that can affect blood pressure and fluid balance. High sodium intake can lead to health issues.

  - Tip: Opt for low-sodium options and use herbs and spices to flavor your food instead of salt.

Calculating Carbohydrates

- **Carbohydrate Counting**

    - Definition: Carbohydrate counting involves tracking the amount of carbohydrates you consume to help manage blood sugar levels.

    - Tip: Use a carbohydrate counting guide or app to help estimate the carbohydrate content of different foods.

- **Exchange Lists**

    - Definition: Food exchange lists categorize foods with similar carbohydrate content. They can help you create balanced meals and manage portions.

    - Tip: Use exchange lists to plan meals and snacks, ensuring that you're getting a variety of nutrients.

- **Glycemic Index**

    - Definition: The glycemic index (GI) measures how quickly a food raises blood sugar levels.

    - Foods with a low GI have a slower, more gradual effect on blood glucose.

    - Tip: Choose low-GI foods to help maintain stable blood sugar levels.

- Portion Sizes

    - Definition: Managing portion sizes is important for controlling carbohydrate intake and maintaining blood sugar stability.

    - Tip: Use measuring cups, a food scale, or visual cues to help control portion sizes and adhere to your meal plan.

www.ingramcontent.com/pod-product-compliance
Lightning Source LLC
Chambersburg PA
CBHW081552250726
48653CB00009B/3402